"In our normal self-critical frame of mind, motivation is something we don't have and ... y taking the cotton out of our ears and shoving motivation into our thick skulls. It rarely works. This book gently asks compassionate and important questions, teaching us how to listen to our own deepest yearnings. Instead of shoving motivation in, this book artfully creates a space for the caring within to step forward and be known. Highly recommended."

—**Steven C. Hayes, PhD**, originator of acceptance and commitment therapy (ACT)

"As we come to understand psychological principles more clearly, it becomes possible for people to learn and apply them in their own lives. In this clearly written book, Michelle Drapkin conveys insights from forty years of research on motivational interviewing (MI) that can be applied to understand and shape your own motivation for change."

—**William R. Miller, PhD**, emeritus distinguished professor of psychology and psychiatry at The University of New Mexico

"This book is a gem! Having worked alongside Drapkin for many years, I have witnessed firsthand her applied science approach to human behavior and to truly helping people. This book combines her knowledge, excellent communication skills, empathy, and wit. Everyone will benefit from this book at their own pace, with limitless potential for positive impact in your life. It's truly wonderful to see such an important contribution to people's lives."

—**Jack Groppel**, internationally recognized pioneer in the science of human performance, and hall-of-fame coach who has authored dozens of books and publications

"The science of MI permeates this book. More importantly, Drapkin permeates this book. What a companion she is! You will get to know a kind, funny, helpful, open, and wise psychologist. She is ready to become your biggest supporter, to accomplish what until now has been so difficult. You will need to do your part, but her presence may make what seemed impossible, quite possible."

—**A. Tom Horvath, PhD, ABPP**, president of Practical Recovery Psychology Group; and author of *Sex, Drugs, Gambling, and Chocolate*

"If you've been working on a goal or change for longer than you'd care to admit, stop whatever you're doing that isn't working, and pick up this book! Drapkin provides a simple, user-friendly, engaging, and insightful process to help you tap into your motivation, reduce interferences, and stay enthusiastic through the change process."

—**Deborah Grayson Riegel, MSW**, communication coach, and author of *Go to Help*

"Behavior change is HARD, especially if you're not one hundred percent sure you want to or can change. Drapkin has come to the rescue with *The Motivational Interviewing Path to Personal Change*. Her guidance is clear, enthusiastic, and most of all…motivating! I highly recommend this book for anyone who is thinking about making a change and could use a wise guide to help show the way."

—**Jill Stoddard, PhD**, author of *Imposter No More*, and cohost of the *Psychologists Off the Clock* podcast

"I've never read a workbook in which the author's voice was more alive in the words. Michelle Drapkin's humor, empathy, and insight suffuse every page of *The Motivational Interviewing Path to Personal Change*. In line with the spirit of MI, she embraces both/and thinking: This is your journey, and she will accompany you every step of the way."

—**Seth Gillihan, PhD**, host of the *Think Act Be* podcast, and author of *Mindful Cognitive Behavioral Therapy*

"What a lovely guide for change! Thank you, Michelle Drapkin, for sitting in the living room with us and guiding us through the changes we hope for in our life. It is rare to get true expertise in the science of change, wrapped in a personal sense of being held and guided through this process we all face day to day: how to move toward the life we truly want."

—**Jeff Foote, PhD**, clinical psychologist; and cofounder of the Center for Motivation and Change (CMC), and the CMC: Foundation for Change

"If you are looking for inspiration for personal movement forward or engagement in values-based living, then *The Motivational Interviewing Path to Personal Change* is the exact book you have been looking for. Michelle Drapkin has written a personable, witty, and thoughtful book about making major changes in life. Drapkin invites readers through focusing, tracking, choosing, and committing to live forward in meaningful and purpose-driven ways. A must-read for genuine and lasting change!"

—**Robyn D. Walser, PhD**, author *The Heart of ACT*; coauthor of *Learning ACT* and *The Mindful Couple*; and assistant professor at the University of California, Berkeley

"Whether you seek sustainable change in your own life, or guidance to design change journeys for others, Michelle Drapkin offers an accessible and engaging road map to get there. I've used MI in my design work for decades; since finishing this book, I'm bursting with energy and ideas to improve how I do it. Change isn't easy, but having *The Motivational Interviewing Path to Personal Change* in your pocket sure helps."

—**Amy Bucher, PhD**, chief behavioral officer at Lirio, and author of *Engaged*

The

Motivational Interviewing
Path to
Personal
Change

The Essential Workbook
for Creating the
Life You Want

Michelle L. Drapkin, PhD, ABPP

New Harbinger Publications, Inc.

Publisher's Note

This publication is designed to provide accurate and authoritative information in regard to the subject matter covered. It is sold with the understanding that the publisher is not engaged in rendering psychological, financial, legal, or other professional services. If expert assistance or counseling is needed, the services of a competent professional should be sought.

The behavior change journey is a common one, and many have walked similar paths. Please know that all patients, friends, and others mentioned as examples in this book are composites of humans I have been lucky to know over the years. Any similarities between what you read and the life you have lived are because we are all in this together and those similarities exist. You are not alone.

NEW HARBINGER PUBLICATIONS is a registered trademark of New Harbinger Publications, Inc.

New Harbinger Publications is an employee-owned company.

Copyright © 2023 by Michelle L. Drapkin
New Harbinger Publications, Inc.
5674 Shattuck Avenue
Oakland, CA 94609
www.newharbinger.com

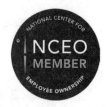

All Rights Reserved

Cover design by Sara Christian

Acquired by Ryan Buresh

Edited by Rona Burnstein

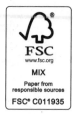

Library of Congress Cataloging-in-Publication Data on file

Printed in the United States of America

25   24   23

10   9   8   7   6   5   4   3   2   1   First Printing

This book is dedicated to all of us working hard out there creating the life we want and all of us working hard to help support other people's change.

Contents

Foreword

Motivational interviewing (MI) has become an evidence-based standard in almost all professions requiring practitioners to establish relationships with their clients, patients, or customers. Actually, this turns out to be most human service enterprises. It seems that if people are involved, MI is often helpful. Or at least that is what the research shows.

It works and that is grand, except that most of us do our living and changing apart from these helping relationships. Even with tough changes—like stopping smoking, losing weight, changing our high-risk substance use—we tend to do it without experts. Without the help of professionals, we try to find a way.

Now, that doesn't mean we do it alone. We talk to friends, family, and coworkers, and share our troubles, sort through options, and get advice—sometimes unwanted. Many times it helps, but not always. Which is why in 2022, the self-improvement industry was valued at $10.4 billion, with self-help books and audiobooks making up about $1.5 billion of that total. We spend a lot of time and treasure on changing "on our own." And while there is science supporting what is being offered, there is also a lot of snake oil being sold, which is why this book is so important.

Dr. Michelle Drapkin has done something remarkable here. She has taken an evidence-based method that involves a particular kind of conversation—one that requires another person to be present—and has created a vehicle for that to happen in a book. We have Dr. Drapkin, an expert in MI, cognitive behavioral therapy (CBT), dialectical behavior therapy (DBT), and behavior change generally, paired with Michelle, the down-to-earth, straight-talking "Jersey Girl" who's been there, done that, and has the love of donuts and a set of workout clothes to prove it. She knows change from the inside out and shares it with warmth, encouragement, and the faith of a scientist-practitioner who believes what the science and her clients have shown her—people can and do change, if we create the right conditions.

Dr. Drapkin, this sharp researcher, trainer, and practitioner, has distilled the essence of MI and placed it into a format where we can both hear her voice and experience her presence, as she gently and compassionately guides us through our change process. She takes the power of this conversational approach and engages us in an internal dialogue with her. The upshot? No cheerleading or false promises here. Instead, we have powerful tools available to harness our motivations for change and a new person in our corner.

This book is a gem. Enjoy your time with Dr. Drapkin. You're in skilled hands and using great tools.

—David B. Rosengren, PhD

President & CEO, Prevention Research Institute

Author, *Building Motivational Interviewing Skills:
A Practitioner Workbook*

Motivational Whaaaaaaat?

People are generally better persuaded by the reasons which they have themselves discovered than by those which have come into the mind of others.

—Blaise Pascal, Pensées

Welcome! If you've picked up this book, it's because you're open to making some change in your life, small or large, to live more of the life you want to live—and you might be struggling a bit to get there. Or you feel like your life needs to change in *some* way, and you're not quite sure how, let alone what path you need to take to get there. That's where motivational interviewing (MI) comes in. MI is an approach specifically designed to help people explore their ambivalence about change, which so often gets in the way of sustainable behavior change. We will use MI together to get you where you want to go, even if you don't know precisely where that is right now.

It might be tough to imagine, but we're going to have so much fun on this journey—your change journey—together; I can't wait! Sure, it's going to be hard and maybe seemingly impossible at times. "Change is hard": I know we've heard that often—it has lots of truth—and the change process can also be exhilarating. Changing behaviors that are important to us is rewarding work. I've devoted my career to helping humans just like you and me make meaningful changes to create the life we want.

Let's start at your beginning. It might help to know more about what brought you here as a starting point to understand where your head is with all this change stuff. What made you pick up this book? Even if you didn't buy it for yourself, why is this book in your hands? What changes are you considering right now? Maybe you already have a few clear targets for change in mind and you want a path forward to get started. Maybe you're dreaming of the life you wish you had—and you feel stuck, again, for the hundredth time, in your path to get there. Or maybe you feel like you just don't know what to do or change. Most people have quite a list of things that they know they want to change, could change, have reasons to change, or need to change. We're humans and we're not perfect.

Let's try to capture why you are here in the first place. We're not looking for you to commit to a specific change target just yet—that will come later, when you're ready. For now, just think about what brought you here, to reading these words and holding this book. If you're feeling up to it, jot some notes down:

_____

_____

_____

This is hard stuff and your change journey likely won't be a straight line. I am not here with overly enthusiastic hoopla to cheerlead you through; that's "toxic positivity" that you won't find here. I know how hard change can be, and my hope for you is that this book helps you start your journey; becomes a tool in your toolbox that helps you get back on that path, over and over; and keeps you on that journey to creating the life you want and being the person you want to be.

But before we get too far into the kickoff party, let's get some basics down together…

What Is Motivational Interviewing?

"Motivational Interviewing" sounds like motivational speaking, eh? I get that a lot. It's pretty different in a lot of ways. I'll explain that more in a sec. For now, what's important to know is that MI is a commonsense approach to behavior change that involves us using what we have inside ourselves—what we value, what is important in our own lives, what we are capable of—to inspire our behavior, rather than feeling pressured to make changes in our lives because of external factors. Which is also to say: MI is about empowering *you*. You are the one making all the choices. Remember, I am not your hypegirl; I'm with you to help you find the power inside yourself to create the life you want and to keep you engaged on that journey. I won't push you; there will be no rah-rah stuff. First because I find that kind of annoying and second because it doesn't work—at least not in the long run. The show *Intervention* makes for good TV watching (lots of drama and emotion), but there are no data to suggest that interventions like those portrayed actually work to change behavior (Kosovski and Smith 2011). An "intervention" is a gathering of people trying to convince or inspire someone to change a behavior that's impacting them and those around them. It's all external motivation for change, and it doesn't do the best job of drawing out the internal, meaningful motivation. In fact, some seemingly well-intentioned people on that show, in using shaming or guilt-inducing statements, might even unintentionally make things worse. Feeling ashamed and bad about yourself is not a helpful place to start a lasting change journey.

In our work together, we're going to do some deep diving into yourself and figure out what drives you forward. What is the gas in your proverbial tank? That's what will keep you on the road even when that road is long and difficult.

Where Are My Manners?

Before we delve too far, you might be wondering…*Who is this person talking to me?* It's a fair question. I am a board-certified clinical psychologist who sees patients in private practice and a behavior scientist who has been working in the MI field for over twenty years. I am a longtime MI trainer and have trained thousands of other clinicians, helpers, and leaders in how to use MI to effect change in their patients and organizations. I simply am passionate about helping people change. I define my sense of purpose as "Better Access to Better Care." I wrote this book to bring to you the tools and resources I share with others every day. You have in your hands my personal recipe for the "secret sauce" of behavior change. Use it wisely (and often).

One way to help you understand the value of MI is by helping you feel how unique and differentiated it is from other approaches. To do that, I'd like to start by telling you about my introduction to it. Sit back, grab a snack, it's story time—a story about an untrained individual who figured out what made MI so distinct (and effective) just by observing it in action. You can also skip this part if it's not of interest to you. One of the most important things to understand in our journey together is that you have choices, lots of choices. This book is intended for you to flip through and find what is of interest to you. There is no "right way" to do anything, including reading this book.

Now, my intro to MI. Between undergrad and grad school, I worked at the University of Pennsylvania in Philadelphia at an addictions research center. I was overseeing randomized controlled trials for addictions and co-occurring conditions (depression and stress/anxiety). My job included working with patients to gather data to use in treatment sessions and research analyses. One of these treatments was called motivational enhancement therapy (MET; Miller 1992), which is a structured version of MI that presents patients with normative feedback—that is, feedback on how they compare to the general population—as part of the treatment process. We would tell patients where they fell in comparison to the population (for example, "70% of the male population in your age range drinks less than you do") or we'd feed them back information they provided to us about perceived consequences of their alcohol or substance use (e.g., how much money they were spending on substance use, how often they missed work or had conflicts with family). The feedback served as a mirror for the patients. It's like when you get blood work from your primary care physician—they tell you how high or low your cholesterol is and if it falls in a "typical range." It's feeding you back information, or data, and putting it in context so you can understand its meaning for you. It was the same for our patients who were struggling to reduce their substance use. We fed them back their data and put it in context for them.

I interviewed patients, created feedback sheets, and listened to recordings of therapists delivering those sessions (to assess their adherence to the therapeutic protocol, not to be nosy!). Remember, I was a wee lass who had just graduated from college—not the trained, sophisticated (maybe even sometimes talented?) psychologist you are hanging out with today. What I heard and observed in those sessions was paradigm shifting. Therapists did not confront patients—no "talking some sense" into them. They did not scare or shame them into change. No "You are ruining your life… you are going to die." Not even "You're hurting your loved ones and yourself." They did not tell them what to do (or not to do) or how to do it (or not do it). They were supportive and collaborative and allowed patients to move at their own pace, reflecting with them on the data in their reports and empowering them to make choices that aligned with their values. The therapists also validated patients' experiences ("It makes sense that this is hard") and helped guide them to what was important to them ("You care about being a good parent, and drinking alcohol doesn't fit with that").

And it worked! Suddenly patients were responding with insights and observations about their data. They were marching toward the change that mattered to them because they were inspired from within, by their own reasons for change—which their therapists had worked *with* them to discover—and not because someone was coercing them. It felt like magic! Patients would share with me their enthusiasm, and you could see it on their faces. They were inspired, engaged, and motivated. It was the opposite of the interventions you see on TV—there was no confrontation, just simple collaboration. I knew almost immediately that not only did I want to help people, I wanted to help people like *that*. It was as much about the process—the *how*—as it was about the *what*. And that is why you and I are here together right now…to get you on your path.

I later wound up on faculty at the University of Pennsylvania doing some of my own MI research and then got to design and lead a national MI/MET training program in the Department of Veterans Affairs (the largest ever in the world to date and one that is still going strong), teaching clinicians across the country how to use MI skills in their work (Drapkin et al. 2016). And now, here we are together doing the stuff that got me so excited all those years ago. Ain't life grand?

Our Journey in This Book

The term "motivational interviewing" doesn't *really* capture what MI is. MI isn't the Tony Robbins of psychotherapy; we're not giving a motivational pep talk or speech. In MI, our stance is that *you* have the motivation within, even if it's a tiny kernel of motivation, or it's hidden deep inside, or you have gotten so far away from it that it's hard to connect with. My job—well, really, our job, together—is to draw that motivation out, help it grow. I believe you have it in there. Everyone wants things to be better in their own lives in their own ways. It's just that many of us haven't discovered how to get there.

Ultimately, MI is a style of interaction, a way of being. That is why the *how* of this book you have in your hands is as important as *what* it contains. If I'm successful, you will feel my partnership and collaboration on this journey—you won't feel me pushing or carrying you. We are walking side by side.

That's also why you'll find a lot of "we" in this book as you read through it. The "we" isn't a royal "we humans." It's me and you: "we." The point of MI is for us to work together, as partners in the change journey. It's also about helping you connect with your values—the things that matter most to you, what drives your life—and move toward a life you believe is worth living. Part 1 of this book, "Engaging," is aimed at getting connected with yourself and consolidating your enthusiasm for this journey. In chapter 1, you'll begin by working to understand your "why" of change—the values that underlie the behavior change you want to achieve—so you can connect on a meaningful level with *why* the change you hope to make is important to you before you really decide on your *what*.

A lot of people start a behavior change process and want to change *everything*. That enthusiasm is awesome, and yet to be most successful, we'll work to focus that energy a bit more. Think of each change you want in your life as a separate dartboard hanging on the wall, each with its own bullseye. If you were throwing darts, you wouldn't know exactly where to aim because there would be so many choices. Your efforts would be diffused across the dartboards. Or you would freeze entirely when you couldn't determine where to start. Choosing a single dartboard to aim at makes it more likely that you'll hit the bullseye. That is the "goal" part of MI, which part 2, "Focusing," is devoted to. Part 2 will help you pick a board and aim at that bullseye! And you can certainly use this book several times as you work your way through the other dartboards.

Chapter 2 will begin turning us to the "what" of your behavior change journey by defining the areas of change you want to work on broadly; and chapter 3 will have us doing some literal target practice—defining your specific goals and truly understanding the path you'll take to meet those goals. Even when individuals come into my practice with a clearly defined goal, I spend time with them clarifying what is important to them. It helps put everything in perspective in a way we don't often do for ourselves.

I've organized this book based on how the science of MI proposes the change process happens—and it isn't linear or prescriptive. The tasks you'll work through in this book are like overlapping stairsteps; you'll go up and down and skip around as you need to. So, you can always skip ahead if you think you have your darts ready. And you can always come back to an earlier chapter if you feel like you went too far ahead. This is your journey, and you choose your own route, speed, and destination, over and over again. (We are in a judgment-free zone, by the way—and just so we're clear, that includes not judging yourself. Change is hard and there will be mistakes and opportunities to learn along the way.)

Part 3, "Evoking," will guide you through tasks involving language and communication so you can move in your desired direction. Chapters 4 and 5 will help you learn how to identify and modify your "change talk"—the way you talk to yourself about change—and how you can use the way you communicate to enlist both other people and your own self in the process of change. These skills will help you continue drawing on that kernel of motivation we talked about, anytime you might need to, and thus keep you on track with the values and goals you'll have settled on—as well as allow you to pivot in or tweak those goals and values whenever you feel you might need to.

That will bring us to part 4, "Planning." You might be curious why we are not starting with planning. But think about it—this very moment, you likely have some of the knowledge and ability to make whatever change you wish to make, and yet you aren't doing it wholly yet. You might even be able to plan like no one's business, and yet you do not execute. It's because the motivation that allows you to execute isn't quite there yet. The work we'll first do in chapters 1 through 5 will help you build that motivation and maintain it. In chapter 6, we'll get to the work of brainstorming and evaluating potential pathways toward change, selecting a starting point, and envisioning your journey—the final steps enabling you to make the change you want to make and keep yourself on track. Finally, in chapter 7, we'll discuss how to maintain the gains you'll have made and prepare you for what to do if old, unhelpful behaviors rear their ugly heads again.

And, well, that's not really the end of the book because, well, behavior change is not really an end—it's a journey. In the epilogue, we'll pull together everything you learned in our journey together in this book and set you up for continued success on your path to living the life you want—knowing you can come back here whenever you need a refresher.

Part of what you will see inherent in the MI approach is what we refer to as "MI Spirit." You know part of this already—partnership and collaboration, and empowerment—the fact that we'll be drawing out both opportunities for change and motivation to change from within you, rather than just having me tell you what to do. I also am coming from the stance that you are smart and capable, and you already know a lot about what we are going to cover in this book. As your helper here, all I can do is help you access what you already have and leverage it to do the good work you want and perhaps need to do—to be who you want to be. That relates to what you are also going to hear a lot of in our work together: acceptance, another component of MI Spirit. This means acceptance of who you are and what you believe in, your values and goals, your abilities to do or not do what you choose, your right to be in charge of your own life. We are all so very amazingly different. In this book, I provide options. My aim is to help you achieve your goals without imposing my values on you, and I am not perfect, even in my highly edited writing, so if I fall short, please know that I support you as you define you.

Finally, my hope is that you feel a ton of compassion—the final piece of MI Spirit—in our journey together. We are here together to help you get to where you want to go. There are no judgments here. This is your life, not mine. Remember, I am not pushy or righteous. I want to help you decide what is best for you. I am not selling you anything. Okay, maybe I am trying to sell you on the idea that you don't need to be sold.

The Science of MI

You might be thinking, *This sounds amazing, but does this really work?* Part of what you will learn about me is that I am part clinician, part trainer, and all scientist. I love data and research. If you will allow me to geek out for a second, I can give you a tiny overview of the massive evidence base supporting MI and the approach we are going to use in this book.

MI was first described forty years ago in the addictions treatment world as an alternative to confrontational approaches (e.g., telling people what to do, how to do it, and scaring them "straight"). By now, enough evidence has been gathered to demonstrate that using an MI-based approach improves outcomes across several behaviors in many different settings. MI has been studied in over 2,000 published research papers and has been shown to increase engagement and effectiveness rates. So, if your helper is trained in MI and uses an MI approach, you are likely to do better (e.g., sleep better, drink less alcohol, smoke less, do better in school, take your medications). The Motivational Interviewing Network of Trainers (MINT), which I am a part of, was established in 1997 and aims to improve the quality and effectiveness of delivery and training of MI. We represent over forty-three countries and thirty-four languages, demonstrating how widely MI is disseminated globally (Frost et al. 2018).

If you want to learn more about MI research, you can follow any of the references provided in the back of the book. My MI colleagues would love for you to read some of their work. And if research isn't your jam, rest assured, MI, the foundation of this book, is backed solidly by a ton of science.

By the way, MI has had great success as an intervention on its own, as a prelude to another form of evidence-based psychotherapy (EBP), and integrated into other EBPs. Some typical EBPs fall under the cognitive behavioral therapy (CBT) umbrella, including traditional CBT for anxiety/ stress, depression, or substance use disorders; dialectical behavior therapy (DBT); and acceptance and commitment therapy (ACT). There are a ton out there (and many more acronyms), and sometimes engaging in treatment isn't as straightforward or easy as it sounds. An EBP might be the thing you need to feel better, and you might need some help engaging and completing one.

You may have picked this book up because your EBP therapist suggested that it could be helpful for you. Sometimes clinicians like myself use MI at the beginning of treatment to help with engagement, to get you started on the right path. When you seem ready, clinicians move toward another EBP as part of the change plan. And, sometimes, when you start an EBP, there are motivational struggles. I sometimes see patients get overwhelmed with homework assignments, for example, even when they know that those assignments are the practice they need to feel better. It can be hard to stay engaged or do the work. That's where the tools and skills we discuss throughout this book can be helpful, too. Staying connected to the "why" even when you are in treatment with a skilled provider is important. Revisiting that "why" regularly helps keep you grounded in what is important and doing the hard work because that's what gets you—and keeps you—on the path to the life you want.

COM-B

Stepping all the way back to behavior science, let me tell you what we know about how people change, in general, and then how that relates to MI. We'll use one of the simpler models to understand how we can make behavior change happen.

When motivation meets capability and opportunity, behavior change happens. We often refer to this as COM-B (capability + opportunity + motivation = behavior change) (Michie, van Stralen, and West 2011). This sounds simple, but let's break it down a smidge. For a behavior to happen, you have to have the capability (technical ability, for example) and opportunity (means, tools, etc.), and your motivation must be higher to do this behavior than another behavior.

Here's a simple example to consider: I am forever trying to be "healthy." Being healthy isn't a behavior; it's a description of a state of being. To get "healthy" (whatever I define as that for myself, my body, my values), I have a slew of behaviors I need to stay engaged with—I need to eat foods that will nourish me, exercise regularly, avoid sweets or eat them in moderation, and so on. Being "healthy" is a complicated business!

Let's pick one piece of that and break it down. If we look at just the behavior of exercising, we can see how the COM-B model comes to life:

Capability (both physical and cognitive/psychological): I need to know how to exercise. Now, I know this may seem silly to some of you athletic humans out there, but I needed to learn how to run—true story. I joined a local running club and had a coach teach me how to run properly (how to hold my body, where my feet should land, how to breathe—who knew how complicated this stuff could be?). I also have a capable body and decent knees (for now!).

Capability is an important component of behavior change—and the reality is most of us have capability down pat. You can eat healthily (i.e., you know which foods are healthy and which aren't, for the most part) or you know how to reduce your substance use. You know how to get to sleep on time. You also most likely know how to floss like a champion. You just don't do it. Knowledge does not lead to behavior change. The knowing how but not doing, my friends, is a motivational deficit. We will get there in a second.

Opportunity (both physical and social): The next big factor, or actually bucket of factors, determining if behavior change is going to happen is if you have the opportunity to achieve the behavior change. In my running example, I *could* have run outdoors part of the year, but I needed access to a treadmill or indoor track when it got too cold or rainy in New Jersey. Even if I knew how to run perfectly, I needed the means to do it. So I also needed proper running attire and shoes.

Opportunity can also relate to social opportunities. Do you have the right social support to make it happen or a social group or system in place to support what you are doing? Think of the more successful weight loss/management programs out there (e.g., WW, formerly Weight Watchers) and the global substance use disorder support networks (e.g., SMART Recovery, Alcoholics Anonymous). They all involve groups of people facilitating behavior change for and with one another.

Or, more simply, do the people around you support the changes you are trying to make? Whenever I'm in my "healthy mode" and trying to kick the more balanced eating into high gear, I remind my husband to *not* bring unhealthy stuff into the house and to cook with less fat. If he isn't supportive in this endeavor, he can take *away* the opportunity for me to be successful. I also need help making the time and space to be healthy and know that my daughter is taken care of (by my husband or other supportive humans). You see how people can contribute to the opportunity bucket of what determines if we make and sustain our behavior change?

And finally, the pièce de résistance, the subject of this whole book…

Motivation: This is where the rubber meets the road. You can be capable and have the means to do a behavior and, at the same time, not yet have the oomph to get yourself going. How many of you have a piece of gym equipment in your home that serves as a clothing rack? I literally have had two treadmills handed down to me over the years that I never used. Ultimately, the other pieces of the model (capability and opportunity) are useless without motivation.

Let's look at COM-B for another behavior. One of my colleagues, Dr. X, texted me this weekend something I often hear: "I want to stop working so hard and enjoy life more." There's a lot to decipher there. Let's start with the behavior of not "working so hard," which can be translated into "working less," and examine each part of the COM-B from that behavioral goal. Is Dr. X capable of working less? Sure, he has the ability to set his schedule, he knows how to use his calendar, and he is capable of communicating with his colleagues and work partners. The opportunity part of COM-B might be one part he could use some help unpacking. Dr. X was reaching out to me, part of his social network, for support, implicitly asking for help or maybe even accountability. He's already thought through whether he can afford to work less (pay essential bills, maintain a certain standard of living) and give up some of his responsibilities, and decided he can. That is all part of the "opportunity" bucket in behavior change. The real challenge for him? Motivation. "Working less" is complicated for Dr. X. You can even hear the conflict in that simple text. He is someone who values hard work and wants to enjoy life more. He is motivated on both sides and needs to navigate what we would call a values conflict. It has him stuck (and because I know Dr. X well, I can share with you that he has been stuck for years "working so hard"). Shifting your motivation to make a change you have both the opportunity and capability to do is hard work, and that is why we are all in this together.

Here is the tricky part: for behavior to be sustainable and lasting, it must come from within. Again, external motivation is sometimes enough to get someone going—and it's rarely enough to keep someone engaged in the change process if there's not an element of motivation that comes from within. Another piece of advice we're often given, "fake it until you make it," can sometimes work because the motivation that's initially a bit forced can convert to something genuine as you experience success. You gain some reinforcement from doing the behavior, or support from the people and circumstances around you, and all of a sudden your mind and body are like *Yeah, this is what I need to do!* And there are also strategies to generate lasting motivation from within. This book will help you connect with your intrinsic (aka internal) motivation and help you stay motivated and create the life you want.

How to Use This Book

All parts of this book are going to give you *options*. For starters, you don't have to read the chapters in order. Some material builds on prior exercises and, even then, I tried to make it so you could go back and forth. Not everyone likes or needs everything. In each chapter you're going to find a series of exercises to do (or not do). If you're up to it, write as much (by hand) as you feel comfortable doing. Studies show that handwriting is more effective than typing for learning purposes. We're going to learn a lot here together, so mark up your book (if you have it in print) or grab a notebook, journal, or some scrap paper if you are willing. It really might make a difference. On the other hand, if you don't like writing, you can try voice memos or other ways that are consistent with how you learn and function. You can also find lots of worksheets and other free tools on the website for this book, http://www.newharbinger.com/51543. (See the very back of this book for more details.)

Odds are you're not going to carry around and reference this book all day long (even if it's an e-book), so you'll find sections labeled "In Your Pocket." These are stops on the journey that offer a pause to take away some insight—for example, to take a picture of something that you can carry "in your pocket" (often, quite literally). Finally, you'll see that I provide a recap at the end of each chapter to remind you of what you accomplished and as a quick reference in case you want to come back.

My hope is that I have succeeded in designing this book to be flexible and functional for *you*. You can flip around or take a more linear approach or do both depending on your mood. It's like a newer version of "choose your own adventure" books. This book is in your hands and is yours. No one is watching. We have a saying in the behavior change field about "meeting someone where they are at." You, also, get to meet yourself where you are at (and be gentle with yourself). If you feel you might need a lesson in that gentleness, visit our Self-Compassion Break in chapter 1.

If someone you view as a helper has suggested you use this book, wonderful! You two can work together on the process. Heck, you can create a little self-change book club with some pals who also want to make some positive changes and work through the exercises together. This book can also be used and shared with professional helpers. I often work through workbooks like this with patients. Therapy is usually one hour a week (if you are lucky), and workbooks like this offer much more opportunity to learn, grow, and practice. Many patients appreciate the effectiveness and efficiency of this approach. Check out the Reading Group Guide at http://www.newharbinger.com/51543 for tips on how to work collaboratively through this book.

That said, many people do not *need* a professional partner in crime to change a behavior. I will try to guide you when that is and isn't necessary. There are times on this journey where it is not advised to go at it alone. While changing is ultimately up to each individual, at times I give patients direct advice on what might be helpful so that they do not continue suffering needlessly.

Finally, if you are here to help someone else change—say, you are a partner, parent, loved one, or even a professional helper—first, thank you! You are a kind human who cares. Second, I hope you already are soaking up some of the tools of the trade. You cannot force someone to do anything. You can, though, be supportive in effective ways. We'll talk a bit more about this later in the book. Hop over to chapters 4 and 5 where we discuss communication specifically.

Ready to Get Started?

Deep breath… That was a lot. It can be both overwhelming and exciting. I want to make sure you know this—behavior change is very possible, and together, we can get you where you want to be, and keep you on that path toward the life you *really* want to be living. You may not even be sure where that is yet—and we will figure it out, and stay in it together, possibly forever. The life you want is possible; this is *your* journey toward it, and this book will help you along the way. I am so glad you are here!

PART 1

ENGAGING

CHAPTER 1

Getting Started: Find Your "Why"

You can't fall if you don't climb. But there's no joy in living your whole life on the ground.

—Unknown

Okay! Getting to the life you want likely requires changing some of your behaviors. And, let's be *really* clear—change is not easy. Sometimes it sounds simple and it's never "easy." While some changes just happen, for most, without any ambivalence, such as going to school, learning to drive, or falling in love, other behavior changes cause us to waffle a bit. It often takes multiple attempts for a meaningful change to "stick," and we all know the hardest part: getting started (Hardcastle et al. 2017).

We're not here to shame you or make you feel bad about where you're at right now. Many of us have been there, right? When we feel so demoralized and down on ourselves that we don't feel like we can get up the gusto to do *anything*, let alone initiate an important behavior change (yet again). I've had patients tell me, sobbing, that they can't believe they are *there* again. Sometimes we make tiny slips back into the old behavior. You might be on a great run of healthier eating, and then you walk into work and there are free donuts, and bam! You are eating one donut, then two, and suddenly, you're experiencing what behavior scientists call the "abstinence violation effect"—and what I like to call a case of the "f*ck its." So, you think, *I've screwed up a smidge—might as well f*ck it and go for broke!* And you choose stuff you might not have chosen for lunch, and so on—and it becomes much harder to get back on that healthy eating path you were on. Ugh. This change stuff is hard business. We don't want you beating yourself up. On the flip side, though, we don't want you feeling so comfortable, or so resigned to your life as it is, that you don't give it a go making the changes you want to make.

And, that is why I'm here, with you, working to help you see your way through it, see *our* way through it. We have to find a "sweet spot"—a direction for change that's robust enough to really *feel* like and *be* a change, yet not so overwhelming that you feel you won't be able to stay consistent or that if you stumble a little it will completely destroy any momentum you've gained. It's this sweet spot that will help get you started and keep you engaged in the change process. And how will we do that?

Self-Compassion

First step…some empathy, compassion for ourselves, and validation: It makes sense this is hard for you. If change were easy, there wouldn't be a million resources (like this one) to help you. And in the moments you struggle with it, you are not alone. There is a universe of us, all out there working on positive change and struggling together. This is what those who study self-compassion call "common humanity." When you're kind to yourself and realistic about the inevitable pitfalls you'll encounter on your change journey, you can move forward toward your goals—and forgive yourself for the lapses along the way. When you show yourself compassion, particularly in moments of struggle, you can step back and feel that change is seriously hard, and there is no magic bullet. It's just the process of applying yourself, with patience and self-compassion, over and over again—using all that's important to you, your values and dreams, and all that you have, like the people who love and care for you, to help you along the way—and doing the best you can from one moment to the next.

For instance, I sit here typing when I probably *should* be spending more "quality time" with my daughter. Being a mindful, attentive parent is something that is super important to me. I could sit here and beat myself up for choosing to write instead—*What is wrong with you, Drapkin?*—or I could turn my empathy and compassion skills on myself, choose to be kind to myself, and move forward toward living my values and reaching toward my goals. *You are writing a book that is consistent with your meaning and purpose, and you can find time later for your other important values, including being a mindful parent. I will "be here now" and then later today do something with my daughter.* That sounds way easier than it is, even for an "expert" like me. And it is possible. By being aware of your values (what really motivates you to make the changes you hope to make), the secrets of behavior change, and how to self-compassionately navigate challenges to behavior change as they arise, you can get to where you want to go.

We're going to talk more about that values stuff in a minute, but first, I want to offer you some skills to deflect the "f*ck its" and the self-criticism, which most of us are quite good at generating! So, let's try out our first skill—turning our kindness, empathy, and compassion, which we can so often and easily deploy with others, on ourselves. This is a tool you'll pull out of your toolbox often—especially when you beat yourself up for, well, being human.

EXERCISE: Self-Compassion Break

Let's start by thinking of a change you are considering making, something you have been meaning to change, wanting to change, something you just haven't gotten right yet. Maybe it's *the* reason you have this book or maybe it's one of many change behaviors you have in mind. Bring it up in your mind and take a moment to see if you can *feel* it in your body, noticing where the struggle and distress show up. Really take a moment to notice the thoughts, the feelings, the sensations that this brings up for you in your mind and your body. (Yes, our bodies often show us when and where we feel stress, pain, or joy. For instance, when I'm stressed, I often notice it in my chest. It feels like I'm sucking air. Right now, even, I just noticed I wasn't breathing.) So, breathe and notice…

Now, with this source of your struggles in mind, turn your kindness to yourself. We can be skilled at being nice and gentle and patient with others, yet we tend to be very hard on ourselves. So, first, take those skills and say to yourself…

This is tough (or *This is a struggle* or *Ooof, this is rough* or *This is stressful* or *This is frustrating* or *This is scary* or whatever works for you).

This is the skill of mindfulness, awareness of the moment, acknowledging how hard this change process can be.

Next, say to yourself, *Struggling is a part of life* or *Other people also struggle with change* or *I am not alone* or *Change is hard for everyone.*

That's what we refer to as "common humanity," acknowledging that this struggle is a part of life for all of us. You are not alone here or ever, really. It feels that way sometimes, and part of this journey is realizing that struggle is part of life. We are all in this together.

I encourage you to remember this and feel this empathy for yourself often and whenever you need it.

The next step is to find a "soothing touch" for yourself. This is *your* soothing touch, so do whatever works for *you*. Try different forms of touch until you find what comforts you. Some people put a hand or both hands over their heart or a soft hand on their cheek or even put both arms across their chest in a "self-hug" kind of gesture. Or, maybe a fist to your chest in a sign of strength. When I first did this, with my hands over my heart, I felt silly—and now I love how it's my secret little way to send myself some kindness and gentleness when I need it, even in a room filled with people. It might feel wonky at first—and, trust me, it can have value.

When you find a personal soothing touch to try out, say to yourself: *May I be gentle with myself* or *May I be kind to myself.*

Also consider asking yourself, *What do I need to hear right now to be gentler and kinder to myself? What would I want from a loving friend or family member? What would be helpful to hear right now?*

Often, while it can be hard to be kind to ourselves, we know exactly what to say to our friends to help them feel better. If you can treat *yourself* the way you'd treat a friend or child or puppy, it can help.

Other ideas:

May I be patient with myself.

May I forgive myself.

May I learn to accept myself and this process for what it is.

Take a moment and observe what this was like for you. What did you notice? What did you learn? Maybe jot some notes down to capture your thoughts and insights if that feels helpful to you.

_____

_____

_____

_____

Consider using this Self-Compassion Break any time of day or night when you are struggling. Remind yourself to notice the moment, be kind to yourself, and remember that you are not alone—struggle like the kind you're feeling is part of life. You may find me with my hand over my heart and you will now know I'm trying to give myself a break, taking a moment to be gentler, kinder to myself so that I can be strong and effective. Rest assured, we will come back to this again when we need to.

That said, maybe the Self-Compassion Break feels too "squishy" for you to seem useful. That's cool. Again, we're here to find tools and strategies that will work for you. And let's align on this point: this journey we are embarking on is not always going to be easy; you'll want to be kind to yourself along the way, even if an explicit Self-Compassion Break doesn't always feel like the right way to practice that kindness.

Story time: How do farmers coax their donkeys to carry their goods to the town square? Well, you can beat Mr. Donkey with a stick to get him moving and keep beating him to keep him moving until he arrives at the town square. After years, that donkey will be beat up, tired, and worn out. Or, you can be sweet to Mr. Donkey: "Come on, fella, let's do this… I know you're tired and I need you to work with me. One step at a time" and give him some carrots to help nourish him and motivate him to keep moving. After years, the donkey you gave carrots to will be happy, healthy, and cared for (and have amazing eyesight).*

You may have heard this carrot/stick metaphor for how we motivate other people (and donkeys). It applies no less to yourself. Even if the outcome is the same whether we use a carrot or a stick, whether we're kind to ourselves or not (that is, the donkey makes it to the town square, and we get to the positive change we are seeking), wouldn't it be awesome-r if we weren't beaten down when we arrived? Use the carrots of kindness, patience, and self-compassion on yourself even when that mean, disparaging voice inside your head—your inner critic—starts grumbling and wants you to use the stick.

Now that we've got the self-compassion foundation laid down, let's move to another helpful foundational component in your change journey: stabilizing yourself.

Stabilizing

We've already established that our work together can be an uphill battle. In fact, odds are it will be a bumpy road. To get started, we need to stabilize. Think about a runner about to dart off in a race. What do they do first? They get in position and stabilize themselves before they launch. In other words, they get grounded. Grounding can mean many things. To start, we are talking about finding the ground below your feet, kind of like that runner.

"Find your feet." Yes. Stop here and let's find our feet. I am typing this from my office and just found my feet (yay for me!). My legs are crossed, so one foot is on the floor, kind of crooked, and the other is up in the air leaning against a filing cabinet. As I find them, I'm realizing I am not super grounded; I don't feel stable. So, let's put both feet on the ground and really notice them. Wherever you are, plant your feet firmly on the floor for a second. Push each toe down, one at a time and *feel* the ground beneath you. Heck, if you are able, stand up and *really* feel the ground.

Once you've found your feet—your sense of stability and presence in *this* moment—see if you can find what grounds you in your change journey: what drives you, what inspires you, what's important to you in your life. This is going to be different for all of us. You may have seen various images depicting what we think change should be—a straight line—and what change really is—a bumpy, up and down journey. My favorite metaphor for the change journey is one of climbing a mountain with all the switchbacks. It's not a straight path upward—it's back and forth until you

---

* Inspired by https://thehappinesstrap.com/donkeys-carrots-sticks/

reach the summit (which you often can't see from the ground). Take a second and think about your mountain. Think about the whole mountain, the journey, and the summit—and the next mountain in the range. Take it all in. What do you notice?

_____

_____

_____

_____

Coming back to what is important to us, why are we even on this journey together? This is an important question to answer—and it might be hard to get to "off the cuff," so we're going to walk through a few exercises together to connect with your "why." As with everything we'll do, there is no right or wrong way to make this happen. You can do all the exercises here or pick one that speaks to you. You can even come on back and do them later, if you feel like you're already grounded enough in your "why." It's up to you because you know what? You are creating the life *you* want and you get to choose.

EXERCISE: Best Self

This is a fun, creative exercise where we use a visualization technique to help us connect with what is important to us. Ready?

Close your eyes and think about when you are your Best Self—most energized, most engaged, living your best life. This might be yesterday or a time in the distant past. Now go ahead, close your eyes (no, really, close them) and imagine.

You back? Okay! Let's try to capture some of what you discovered. Jot a few notes below. Who is with you when you feel like your Best Self? What are you doing? Where are you? Notice the stories you are telling yourself…including any "Yes, but" ones (e.g., "*Yes* I am most energized when I am working out consistently, *but* I can't find the time). Notice them and focus on the whole scene with you as your Best Self. Here is mine:

Strong, in charge/control, surrounded by my family (schnauzers, human kid, awesome partner), looking and feeling healthy. I am working on my life's purpose/passion and helping people by doing therapy, writing, and posting fun, helpful stuff to social media, and I am somewhere in my town surrounded by my neighbors. I am leading my best life…

Your turn:

_____

_____

_____

_____

How hard or easy is this for you to do? Here are some words that might help you describe your Best Self:

Assertive	Gentle	Rational
Brave	Grateful	Reliable
Caring	Hardworking	Resilient
Compassionate	Healthy	Responsible
Confident	Honest	Romantic
Educated	Kind	Sensitive
Efficient	Loyal	Serious
Empathetic	Mature	Smart
Flexible	Motivated	Strong
Focused	Open-minded	Sweet
Friendly	Patient	Thoughtful
Funny	Practical	Trustworthy
Generous	Proud	Witty

Now comes the really creative version of this. We are going to draw (yes, draw) our Best Self. Don't panic if drawing is not your jam; I am terrible at art. My creative juices almost never land in the art, crafty realm. It's okay. This is just an opportunity to get a visual. So before you close the book and run away if you, too, are not an artist, let me share my Best Self masterpiece:

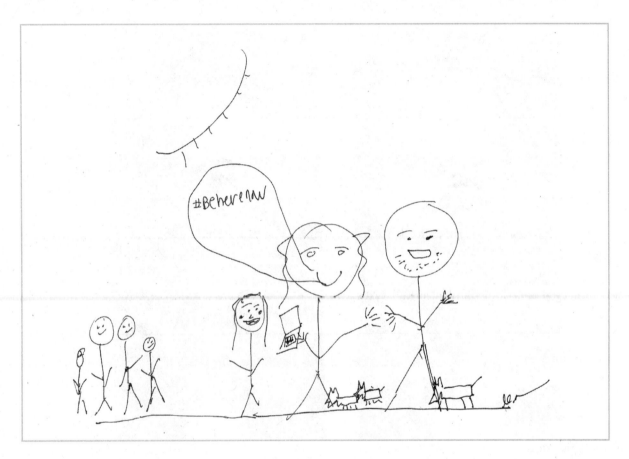

Check out this awesomeness. There is me in the middle, high-fiving my husband, whom I consider my partner in every sense of the word. You also see my schnauzers (don't judge the quantity), my human kid smiling bright and wide, and representative members of our community hanging out in the sunshine with us. And, yes, that is a laptop (not drawn to scale because I am not a skilled artist) with me, just like it is right now as I'm writing this book (incidentally one of the adorable schnauzers is staring at me, one is napping close by, and one is licking his paws, warmed on the radiator), while my husband sits near me on the couch (the human kid is still snoozing in bed). This drawing of my Best Self helps bring that self to life and helps me notice when I am in and when I am out of it.

Okay. Now that I have outed myself with my awesome artwork, it's your turn. Look back at what you wrote above and think about who you are at your best and what that looks like for you. This, like everything in this book, is for *you*, so make it yours. Draw a stick figure or make it super fancy. Heck, put stickers on it. You can even use glitter if you want; the book and I won't judge you. You do *you* and bring your Best Self to life.

Now, one final step: drafting a Best Self statement. Take a look at what you wrote above and your drawing and pull it all together into a single sentence; feel free to use a semicolon and make it a long sentence (it's a trick us academic writers have been using for years—check out the parentheses usage, too!).

I am my Best Self when

_____

_____

_____

_____

_____

_____

Alright, time to take a step back. Are you noticing gaps between your Best Self and where you are now? Good! Those gaps are opportunities to turn your Best Self into more of a consistent reality.

Check out how this plays out in my life:

I am typing this while sitting in the corner of a gym while my daughter has basketball practice. I look up occasionally to observe her, and I am not really present. In fact, I sat myself behind a table to protect my precious laptop from a rogue basketball. I am aware that I am not really aware. I *should* close my laptop and be present. That would be more consistent with my Best Self. Or, maybe I could run laps around the gym while she is running drills, to keep up with my values of fitness and health. And here I am, writing a book that I hope will help us all stay on track with our positive behavior change, and realizing there are still opportunities for myself. What if, instead, I left the laptop at home and was more present at her practice? Or what if I helped the coaches as a way to be part of my community, which is something I value? Also, I don't know much about basketball, and this way, I might lean into my values of *growing and learning (and fitness). There are several ways to navigate what I identify as a values conflict that is keeping me from my Best Self.*

REFLECTION PITSTOP. Now let's take a moment to zero in on any gaps you might have noticed in your life and identify opportunities to narrow or close them. Allow your mind to be in the present moment.

Be here now... And breathe, and know you are breathing.

And while you are here, where are you? How close are you to your Best Self—your vision for who you really want to be? What opportunities are there to close the gap?

Jot a few notes here about your own opportunities you noticed: _____

_____

_____

_____

We'll come back to these opportunities because that's where we can focus our change. First, though, let's dig into this a little deeper by exploring our values. I have to admit that this is my *favorite* thing to do with patients! I love values work! Now, let's roll up our sleeves and get down to what is important at your core—your values.

Values, as described in MI and other related therapeutic approaches, are a curious concept, so let's define them together before we move on.

What Are Values?

In MI, we think of values as the building blocks to our meaning and purpose. They are the components of what drive our behaviors. Values are deeply held beliefs about what is important to you. We are going to spend some time identifying them because they help guide what we do, or at least they *can* guide what we do. You may have even wound up here reading this book because you noticed (mindfully or not) that you were *not* acting in line with your values; that the way you live your life day to day doesn't really reflect what's most meaningful to you. Think about the Opportunities exercise above, which points to the discrepancies that may exist between your Best Self and where you are right now. Implicitly, your values helped you figure that out.

As we're defining "values," one point is especially important: values are different from goals. Goals are specific things we want to accomplish. If living life is like driving a car, goals are the destinations we drive toward and how we will know if we have arrived wherever it is we want to be. Values, on the other hand, are connected to the "why" behind our driving—why we're even driving, or moving toward a particular goal, in the first place. Which is to say, our goals are informed by our values, and they're not the same as values. Through our work together, you'll shift toward creating a life based on your values and not just focused on goal achievement—it will help you have a more fulfilling journey toward achieving your goals.

Take a moment to think about what your values might be. And where they might come from. Our values derive from lots of different places: our rearing (our parents, our community, our extended family); our education (what we have learned in school and life); our religious or other affiliations; and more. The cool thing about values is that they're shared concepts, meaning you likely share values you hold with others—and yet the mix of which ones are most important to you is incredibly individualistic and unique. Here, I offer a couple of exercises to help you more clearly assess your values. You get to choose which exercise you want to do—or do all of them—up to you.

EXERCISE: Identifying and Prioritizing Your Values

Our first opportunity to assess your values is a classic MI exercise referred to as the Personal Values Card Sort (Miller et al. 2001), which I have adapted for our use here.

Step 1: Below you'll find a list of values, and columns to note whether each value is Not Important, Somewhat Important, or Very Important. You are going to cruise through the values listed and decide which category each falls into for you. There's also a blank spot in case the list doesn't capture a value that is meaningful to you.

Aim to have about ten values in the Very Important category. You'll probably feel like everything is very important. It might be—and yet it can't all be very important at the same time. Ultimately, life is about maneuvering competing values. You saw that in my example above. When I was at my daughter's basketball practice, I was writing parts of this book, which is super meaningful and aligned with one of my values, Contribution, the ability to contribute something of real meaning to others and the world around me. I was also struggling with another of my values, Family, which was competing with my Contribution value. So having clarity regarding our most important values and how they relate to one another is important.

Try to think about what is important to you (not me, not your mother, not society, *you*). Again, while values in general are held by many people, they are also, by their definition, individualistic. My values vary even from my husband's. Sure, our values are aligned (mostly!), and they are also different. My values are ultimately *mine*.

Ready? Let's do this! Look at each value below and note whether it is Not Important (N), Somewhat Important (S), or Very Important (V) for you. You can download this Values Table from the website for this book, http://www.newharbinger.com/51543. Or, if you're more of a tactical person, you can download and print a "card" version from the website. Both offer the same values, so use whichever feels like a better fit for you.

VALUES TABLE

N, S, OR V?	VALUE: DESCRIPTION	N, S, OR V?	VALUE: DESCRIPTION
	ACCEPTANCE: to be accepted as I am		INDUSTRY: to work hard and well at my life tasks
	ACCURACY: to be accurate in my opinions and beliefs		INNER PEACE: to experience personal peace
	ACHIEVEMENT: to have important accomplishments		INTIMACY: to share my innermost experiences with others
	ADVENTURE: to have new and exciting experiences		JUSTICE: to promote fair and equal treatment for all
	ATTRACTIVENESS: to be physically attractive		KNOWLEDGE: to learn and contribute valuable knowledge
	AUTHORITY: to be in charge of and responsible for others		LEISURE: to take time to relax and enjoy
	AUTONOMY: to be self-determined and independent		LOVED: to be loved by those close to me
	BEAUTY: to appreciate beauty around me		LOVING: to give love to others

Not Important (N), Somewhat Important (S), or Very Important (V)

N, S, OR V?	VALUE: DESCRIPTION	N, S, OR V?	VALUE: DESCRIPTION
	CARING: to take care of others		MASTERY: to be competent in my everyday activities
	CHALLENGE: to take on difficult tasks and problems		MINDFULNESS: to live conscious and mindful of the present moment
	CHANGE: to have a life full of change and variety		MODERATION: to avoid excesses and find a middle ground
	COMFORT: to have a pleasant and comfortable life		MONOGAMY: to have one close, loving relationship
	COMMITMENT: to make enduring, meaningful commitments		NONCONFORMITY: to question and challenge authority and norms
	COMPASSION: to feel and act on concern for others		NURTURANCE: to take care of and nurture others
	CONTRIBUTION: to make a lasting contribution in the world		OPENNESS: to be open to new experiences, ideas, and options
	COOPERATION: to work collaboratively with others		ORDER: to have a life that is well-ordered and organized
	COURTESY: to be considerate and polite toward others		PASSION: to have deep feelings about ideas, activities, or people
	CREATIVITY: to have new and original ideas		PLEASURE: to feel good
	DEPENDABILITY: to be reliable and trustworthy		POPULARITY: to be well-liked by many people
	DUTY: to carry out my duties and obligations		POWER: to have control over others
	ECOLOGY: to live in harmony with the environment		PURPOSE: to have meaning and direction in my life
	EXCITEMENT: to have a life full of thrills and stimulation		RATIONALITY: to be guided by reason and logic

Not Important (N), Somewhat Important (S), or Very Important (V)

N, S, OR V?	VALUE: DESCRIPTION	N, S, OR V?	VALUE: DESCRIPTION
	FAITHFULNESS: to be loyal and true in relationships		REALISM: to see and act realistically and practically
	FAME: to be known and recognized		RESPONSIBILITY: to make and carry out responsible decisions
	FAMILY: to have a happy, loving family		RISK: to take risks and chances
	FITNESS: to be physically fit and strong		ROMANCE: to have intense, exciting love in my life
	FLEXIBILITY: to adjust to new circumstances easily		SAFETY: to be safe and secure
	FORGIVENESS: to be forgiving of others		SELF-ACCEPTANCE: to accept myself as I am
	FRIENDSHIP: to have close, supportive friends		SELF-CONTROL: to be disciplined in my own actions
	FUN: to play and have fun		SELF-ESTEEM: to feel good about myself
	GENEROSITY: to give what I have to others		SELF-KNOWLEDGE: to have a deep and honest understanding of myself
	GENUINENESS: to act in a manner that is true to who I am		SERVICE: to be of service to others
	GOD'S WILL: to seek and obey the will of God		SEXUALITY: to have an active and satisfying sex life
	GROWTH: to keep changing and growing		SIMPLICITY: to live life simply, with minimal needs
	HEALTH: to be physically well and healthy		SOLITUDE: to have time and space where I can be apart from others
	HELPFULNESS: to be helpful to others		SPIRITUALITY: to grow and mature spiritually

Not Important (N), Somewhat Important (S), or Very Important (V)

N, S, OR V?	VALUE: DESCRIPTION	N, S, OR V?	VALUE: DESCRIPTION
	HONESTY: to be honest and truthful		STABILITY: to have a life that stays fairly consistent
	HOPE: to maintain a positive and optimistic outlook		TOLERANCE: to accept and respect those who differ from me
	HUMILITY: to be modest and unassuming		TRADITION: to follow respected patterns of the past
	HUMOR: to see the humorous side of myself and the world		VIRTUE: to live a morally pure and excellent life
	INDEPENDENCE: to be free from dependence on others		WEALTH: to have plenty of money
	Other Value Not Listed above:		WORLD PEACE: to work to promote peace in the world

Not Important (N), Somewhat Important (S), or Very Important (V)

Now, take a step back and notice what it was like for you to go through that exercise. For some people, it's hard to *just* put ten or so values in the Very Important category. It feels "bad," like you're choosing a favorite child or leaving too much out by focusing on only ten important values. The challenge is understandable; it's also part of the exercise. In the end, the values exercise is an opportunity to sit back and think about what is *really* important and how you let those most important things rise to the top. And sadly, not everything can be that important. Feeling that way is often how we get ourselves into trouble by not prioritizing, which we'll get to in Step 2.

Look closely at what you put in the Very Important category. Are there only ten-ish in that category? If not, try to chop it down a smidge more.

Here's a version of mine I did with cards a couple of years ago. Notice that I was not successful at getting down to ten. We can't all be perfect and orderly. I guess it's ironic that Order is the bottom value here. I also "cheated" and put Family, Loved, and Loving together, treating them as a single integrated value. It's okay. You know why? Because they are *my* values.

AUTONOMY

to be self-determined and independent

7

LOVED

to be loved by those close to me

48

FAMILY

to have a happy, loving family

25

LOVING

to give love to others

49

CARING

to take care of others

9

COMFORT

to have a pleasant and comfortable life

12

CONTRIBUTION

to make a lasting contribution
in the world

15

GROWTH

to keep changing and growing

34

MINDFULNESS

to live conscious and mindful of the
present moment

51

HUMOR

to see the humorous side of myself
and the world

40

GENUINENESS

to act in a manner that is true
to who I am

32

ORDER

to have a life that is well-ordered
and organized

57

Step 2: Now let's focus on those Very Important values. In the table below (also available at http://www.newharbinger.com/51543), sort them from 1 to 10 (ish), with 1 representing the most important value in the Very Important list, and 10 the least important. This is probably the hardest part of this exercise, so if you run into difficulty figuring out how to sort the values, have some self-compassion.

Often patients ask, "Should I rank based on how I am living my life or how I feel like I *should* be living my life?" What this question is really getting at is the realization that often, if someone dropped in and observed our behaviors, they might get the wrong idea about what is important to us, what we value. What we end up doing day to day may not always speak to our values in quite the way we might hope. Much like the Opportunities exercise above, this exercise is a chance to begin understanding where you are versus what you think or feel is most important to you. And it's okay if either of those two, where you are now and what you think or feel you most value, ends up shifting over the course of the activity or this book or life. It's all part of the process.

Once you've ranked your top ten values, ponder the questions in column 2 for each value. Then, in column 3, note how aligned your life is with each value, from 0 (not at all aligned) to 10 (couldn't be more aligned).

Top Ten Very Important Values

VERY IMPORTANT VALUE	WHAT DOES THIS VALUE MEAN TO YOU? HOW DOES IT SHOW UP IN YOUR LIFE?	HOW ALIGNED IS YOUR LIFE WITH THIS VALUE? 0–10
#1		
#2		
#3		
#4		
#5		
#6		
#7		
#8		
#9		
#10		

Note: There are a couple of extra lines just in case.

REFLECTION PITSTOP: OPPORTUNITIES PART DEUX. What did you observe as you went through this exercise? Just like you might have done above with the Best Self exercise, what gaps did you notice between where you currently are, in terms of living your life according to what you value most, and how you want to be living? And what opportunities might you have uncovered to narrow that gap? Capture some of your thoughts and feelings here.

_____

_____

_____

_____

_____

_____

_____

IN YOUR POCKET: Here is the real pro tip: write down your top ten values and take a picture of them. That way, they'll always be with you, right on your phone. You can review it over and over again when you are faced with tough (or even simple) decisions and ask yourself, Is this in line with my values? You can even make it the background on your phone's home screen. This way you can keep your values top of mind as guides for the life you want to live and the kind of person you want to be.

EXERCISE: Bullseye Values Exercise (Harris, 2019)

This is an exercise to get at your values in a different way. You can skip it or use it to take a deeper or different look at the values you just identified. Or, maybe this feels like a better fit for you to discover those values than the values exercise above. The Bullseye is also available at http://www.newharbinger.com/51543.

This exercise uses the image of a dartboard (see below) divided into four meaningful domains of life—work/education, leisure, relationships, and personal growth/health—to help you think about your values and how you might be living them now. First, write down your values in these four areas of life. Again, these are your values, not mine, not your partner's, not your neighbor's. We are trying to connect to your more general life directions, not specific goals. So, think deep and broad here. Think about your values as if there were nothing in your way, nothing stopping you from living them. What's important? What do you care about? And what do you want to drive toward? Values indicate how you want to live your life overall, over time. For example, my goal today is to exercise for twenty minutes; the related value is health and wellbeing, which also ladders up to many other values across domains.

Ready for a dive deep into these areas? Let's start!

1. **Work/Education:** Think about your work, your career, your education/schooling, any kind of skills or knowledge that you want to develop or already are. This can also include related areas like volunteer or pro bono work. How do you want to show up in these settings, with your colleagues, to your customers, direct reports, managers, professors, fellow students? How would you want someone to describe you? What do you want to be really "expert" at (what skills do you want to develop)? Jot some notes down here about your values in this domain.

   _____

   _____

   _____

2. **Relationships:** Here, think about all kinds of relationships—romantic/intimate ones, friends, children, parents/other family, coworkers, neighbors. What kinds of relationships are important to you? How do you want your important people to describe you? And what are you still working on or wanting to develop in those relationships? Notice what values are important to you in your relationships and take a few notes below.

   _____

   _____

   _____

3. **Personal Growth/Health:** This is a big one—broadly, what is important to you as a human? Think about how creative or not creative you are, your spiritual or religious beliefs, your life skills, what drives you. Also dive into your values related to health and wellbeing. Think about how those all come together, and capture some values below.

_____

_____

_____

4. **Leisure:** Now the "fun" one. Spend some time mulling over how you "play," chill out, relax, have fun, all of it. Think about your hobbies and any activities you do (or wish you did more often) that are meaningful to you and why. Capture the values associated with these.

_____

_____

_____

The bullseye: Read through the values you wrote down above, then make an X in each of the four quadrants of the dartboard to indicate where you are at this very moment. An X in the bullseye (center of the board) means that your life is fully aligned with your values in that area of your life. An X far from the bullseye means that something is a bit off between your values and how you are living your life.

Here is what the markings might look like for someone whose relationships are closely aligned to their values while their work/education and personal growth/health domains are somewhere in the middle. Leisure is "out there," meaning they've lost touch with their values. Remember my colleague Dr. X? This sounds like him in some ways, right?

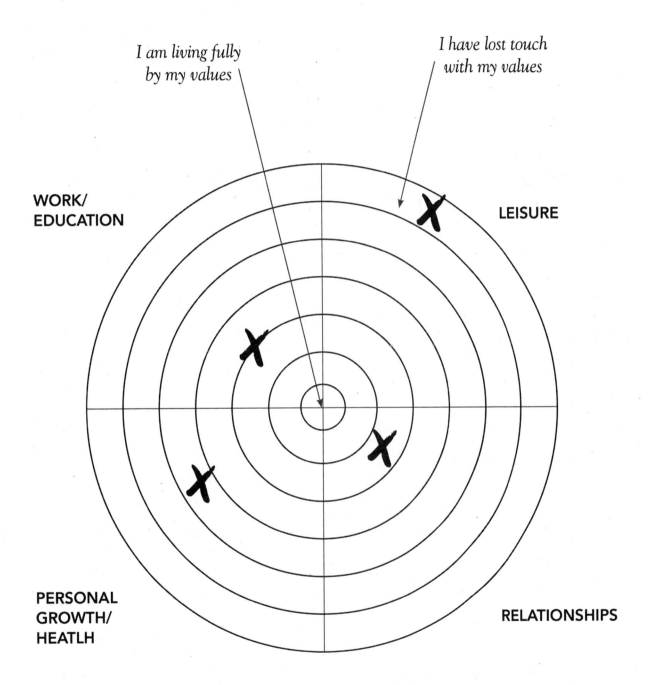

Now your turn. How aligned is your life with your values? Place your Xs.

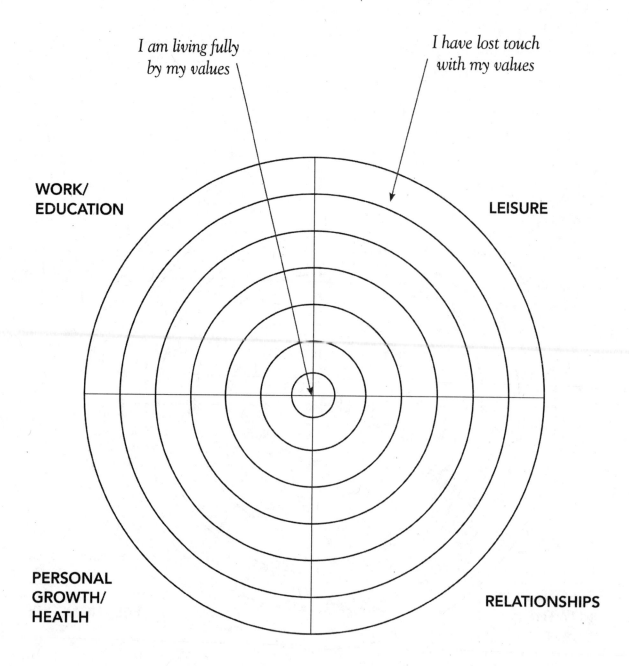

I am living fully by my values

I have lost touch with my values

WORK/ EDUCATION

LEISURE

PERSONAL GROWTH/ HEATLH

RELATIONSHIPS

REFLECTION PITSTOP: OPPORTUNITIES REVISITED. This is our third time taking a moment to stop and think about opportunities, possibilities, the road ahead of us. You have grounded yourself and explored your Best Self and your values (two ways, I might add). What are some opportunities the Bullseye Values Exercise brought up for you? Which domains are you kicking butt in, and which might be suffering a bit right now? Where are the opportunities to grow?

_____

_____

_____

_____

That was a lot of work figuring out our "why" from a variety of angles. You may have chosen to do some of the activities and left others behind. Either way, they're always there for you to visit or revisit. Perhaps you were already sure of what you want to change and why, and these exercises were helpful to reinforce all of that; or maybe you discovered some new directions in which you might like your life to go. Now that we're a little more grounded in our "why," let's rejoin the journey and wrap up this chapter with some acceptance.

Radical Acceptance

Positive behavior change is hard. Odds are you'll be working against some well-worn habit pathways as you work to create new ones. It's not impossible; it's just not easy. And owning the "hard"ness is going to help you in the long run. Notice this is *acceptance*, not *resignation*. In the times when things feel bad or hard, we're not just laying down and "taking it." No, we are accepting that this is how it is. We sometimes call this "radical acceptance" because we are taking a clear, radical stance of acceptance.

I know...this might be tough to swallow, but here it goes...change is an ongoing, lifelong process that requires vigilance and maintenance. Ugh. That sounds icky or grueling. And yet it can be empowering when we step back and really own it. You are going to work hard at changing your behavior, and if you stop working (let your guard down), your old behaviors will creep back in. This explains why I am on this journey with you. I am still *in it* and always will be. Here is what happens to me: I think, *I've got this…look at me, strong and healthy*. And then I begin to lose sight of how my behaviors are connected to (literally responsible for) the way I feel. Other parts of life get in the way, and I stop working out as often, loosen up my vigilance on what I'm eating, and start to slip. And I catch myself over and over again.

Here is the good, empowering news: as you work on maintenance—the things you need to do to continue making the change you've committed to—it becomes "less work." That is, newer behaviors become automatic habits you do without thinking about it (just like the older ones were before). And as that happens, it becomes most important to work on finding reinforcers to keep yourself engaged in the change cycle so that these increasingly automatic habits remain a sustainable part of your routine. Try out the Change Master of the Past exercise in chapter 2 to reconnect with some of the skills you already have on board. And, never fear, we will spend time working through these maintenance skills in chapter 7.

Moving Forward

Here's a recap of what we learned and did in this chapter:

- Discovered the Self-Compassion Break, a tool to be kind to ourselves when we are struggling

- Found our feet (aka got grounded) so we can hold steady as we get ready to launch

- Connected with our Best Self to give us a clearer vision of who we want to be

- Explored our values to help us really lean into our "why" and connect with what is important to us

- Discovered some opportunities by looking at the gaps between where we are and where we want to be

- What else? What are you taking away from this chapter?

_____

_____

_____

You can use the skills you learn in this book—self-compassion, grounding, values clarification, and many more to come—over and over again to help keep you engaged in your change journey.

In the next part of the book, you'll use your "why" and really connect to which changes are important (maybe even urgent)—the "what." We will continue to work together to determine what specific changes you want to make in your life. Reasons change a smidge over time while your values, your beliefs, who you are at the core are likely to hold steady. It's important to connect deeply with that. Let's hop over to chapter 2 and get started!

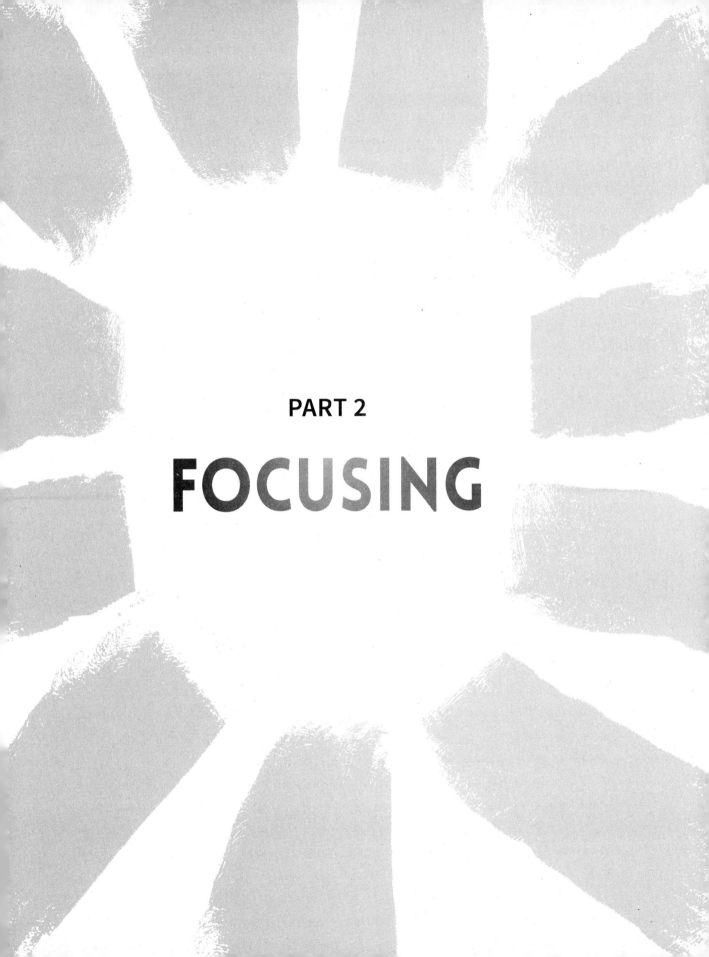

PART 2

FOCUSING

CHAPTER 2

Knowing What You Want to Change

Every action you take is a vote for the type of person you wish to become.

—James Clear

If you are joining me here after completing some of the exercises in chapter 1, I hope you are jazzed and feeling connected to what is important to you. Or maybe you're a little nervous or worried, wondering how you've gotten to where you are in life and how you're going to get back on track with where you want to be. Ultimately, when you're super excited and zoom off into Changeland without a true destination in mind, you can run into trouble. Ever venture out to have lunch without a clear idea of where you want to go, or what you want to eat, and end up driving aimlessly for a while, hungry and frustrated? Or sit down to watch "something" and wind up scrolling through one streaming service after another only to end up disappointed and unsatisfied? Yeah, that is no bueno. It's not a great way to start a change journey either. Even if you're excited, motivated, and engaged at the beginning, you'll quickly peter out without a clear direction. On the flip side, if you're feeling nervous or daunted, the process of really dialing down on a place to start, as we'll do in this chapter, might be clarifying and comforting for you. So, we start by looking for the "what"—our target—in an MI task we call "focusing."

EXERCISE: Exploring Your "What"

Here is the good news. You already laid a lot of the groundwork for this exercise in chapter 1. And, if we are honest, you probably picked up this book with a general "what" in mind—a sense of the change you want to make. Go back and look at what you captured in the introduction. What we're doing here is starting to solidify the exact, concrete change you want to make as a starting point toward your values and your Best Self. So, first step, meander back and look at your values and/or your Best Self. Even if you didn't complete those exercises, take a moment and really connect with what is important to you, who you want to be.

For me, this is "big picture," high-level stuff like:

I want to be present with my family. I want to be healthy and energized. I want to contribute—to my family, my community, the world. I don't want to mess up (I am a smidge of a perfectionist). And I want to be in charge of how I do all of that. Oh, yeah, and I want to have fun and maybe make people laugh (at me or with me—doesn't really matter) along the way.

When I work through this activity with patients, so many different things show up. A few want to be more available for their families, which might mean working less (like Dr. X). Others want to procrastinate less, which can mean working more or more efficiently. People often want to feel less anxious and be more engaged in their lives and want to feel less depressed and enjoy life more. Maybe they want to spend more time with people they care about or engage in more hobbies. I often work with people who are trying to reduce alcohol and other substance use or change other unhelpful habits, everything from smoking cigarettes to biting nails to curbing social media usage.

Now it's your turn. Jot down some notes that will connect you to the feeling of what is important to you and to what you might have captured in chapter 1. This is a place to think about what matters to you and what path you might choose to create the life you want. Think of forest-level stuff. Don't get caught up in a corner of the forest thinking too much about one type of tree.

_____

_____

_____

_____

_____

Honesty time. Look in the mirror, literally or figuratively, whatever works for you. Where are you *now*, today, in relation to what you noted above? Where do you see the biggest gaps between what is important to you/who you want to be and where you are right now, here today? What are you doing well and feeling fully aligned with? Take a moment and look at your daily life. Hey, even pull out your calendar and do an audit of your time. Where are you spending most of your time, investing your energy? How does it match up to what is important to you? How often in your life do you feel animated and engaged?

_____

_____

_____

Step back and take in all the "data" you have collected here and in chapter 1. What do you *feel* are your biggest opportunities for change at this moment? What does your heart say? What does your mind say? Let's pull it all together into a few categories, or, as we referred to them earlier, buckets. What are your big change buckets?

Let's start by naming those buckets. Don't worry about how big or small these buckets are or finding the perfect name for them. This is just a starting point, a step on the journey—which is *your* journey, so there is no right or wrong here, no one way to do this.

Here is what I came up with for my big buckets:

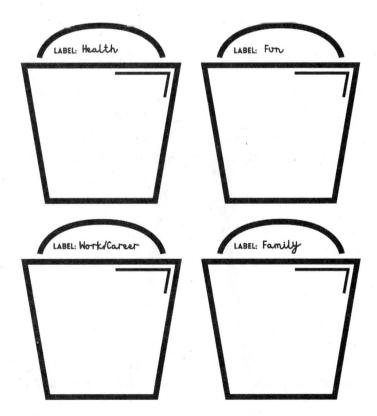

Now, take a second and think about what is important to you and how to bucket those things. You don't need four buckets. You can have any number of buckets. These are here as a place for us to begin. Heck, if you don't like the idea of buckets, use whatever visual or metaphor works best for you. We are stepping into the change journey by first figuring out which "neighborhoods" of change we want to drive toward.

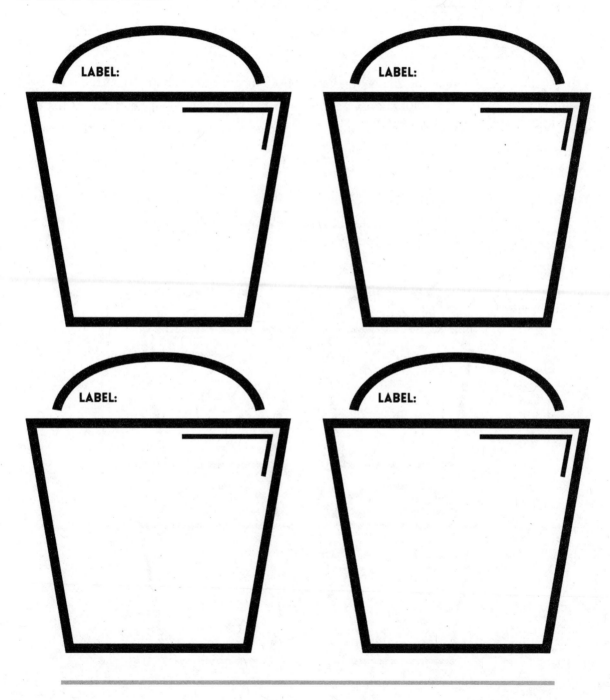

This is a good start. And a great way to look ahead. Let's shift and look back for a moment. At this point in the journey, sometimes people get overwhelmed, dismayed, maybe even frustrated. As they contemplate what they want to be different in their lives, their minds start to look for a path forward, and they wonder how achieving that path will be possible. Maybe right now you are even tempted to toss this book aside and give up. Notice that, be gentle with yourself, find your feet, take a Self-Compassion Break (chapter 1), and let's visit with Past You for a moment.

EXERCISE: Change Master of the Past

Sometimes we start a change process feeling kind of hopeless. The reality is we are often "past life" change masters. Think about this for a second—you likely have changed *something* in your life at some point, even if it felt like something small. Maybe you finally managed to remember to floss or brush your teeth at night, after struggling to stay on top of that routine in the past, or remembered to turn off the lights before you leave the house. Or, maybe you finally got good at budgeting and paying bills. These are all behavior changes. Sure, they may not seem as life changing as other changes you might be considering, and the basic principles are pretty much the same. In a second, you will think this through for yourself. For now, here is a peek into my past change master:

> When I was in grad school, I lost seventy-plus pounds because my life had started to feel unmanageable and unhappy as an unhealthy human. And, do you know what I just remembered? I didn't step foot in the gym until I had lost about forty of those pounds. I was too ashamed and afraid to. At some point, I gathered the courage and went to the Rutgers gym, signed up for personal training and got into a routine, made gym friends, and found a stronger, more confident version of myself. My mind keeps reminding me that I haven't been in a gym in nearly three years and that I weigh more than I "should"—and I bring my mind back to this exercise. Past me has kicked butt in the change arena, and future me can, too!

Your turn! Close your eyes for a moment and think: What have you had some success changing in the past? What positive change have you succeeded at for any amount of time? Again, this doesn't have to be some giant change. It can be something small. My other big accomplishment in life relates to flossing. I hate flossing. I figured out what I really disliked was wrapping floss around my fingers and feeling like I was shoving my whole fist in my mouth to floss. At some point, I had an honest conversation with a dental hygienist. First, I shared with her what I do for a living—that I train health care providers to have more effective conversations about behavior change with their patients. Then I explained how I do that, including the fact that research has shown that giving people choices when they're trying to make a change in their lives is a powerful tool to make lasting changes—people get to choose their own path. She then helped me see that there were options around flossing. I discovered two things that day. First, while not equivalent, a water flosser is a better option than nothing (and is a fun mini power washer on your gums and the sink). Second, there are tools to make flossing easier, including small pre-threaded flossers, which now have me flossing more often than never.

Here's the thing. You are not me. We need to understand what works for you, what tools and skills you have onboard and which you might need to develop, and what steps you can take to work *with* yourself, rather than *against* yourself, as you try to make the changes you hope will last. So it's your turn to visit with your past self. Allow your mind to wander back in time to a moment when you were successful at making a change...

If you're willing, close your eyes for a moment.

No, really, if we are going to do this exercise together, close your eyes and think about your internal change master and all those changes you've made, small and big. Connect with it all.

Eyes open? Fill out as much of this worksheet as you can, and let's take a look at what you know already:

Positive behavior change: What behavior(s) did you change previously?

_____

How similar or different was that change compared to what you're thinking of changing now?

_____

_____

Which bucket does the past change fall in?

_____

_____

How did you make the change happen? Did you need to learn a new skill?

_____

What worked to support your change?

_____

_____

Why?

_____

What didn't work for you?

_____

_____

Why?

_____

Who was instrumental in supporting your change?

_____

What did you learn from this past change experience, if you had to boil it all down?

_____

If you could go back in time, what advice would you give your past self? What would you do differently?

_____

_____

_____

_____

And in which ways did you knock it out of the park? What parts of your past change process would you implement again?

_____

_____

Other insights or observations?

_____

_____

_____

Ambivalence

Because it has likely already shown up in some subtle and maybe not-so-subtle ways, it's important for us to talk about a completely normal part of the change process—ambivalence. Ambivalence is a big, yet important word. "Ambi" means two and the "valence" part stands for feeling—so "ambivalence" means feeling two (or more) ways about something. Ambivalence about change is normal and, frankly, expected. We often feel two ways about a ton of things. For example, you might feel two ways about being a parent. I do! I love my daughter. She is amazing on so many levels…*and* being a parent has changed my life in many ways, not all of them awesome. I'm busier, I'm more tired, and I have a ton to juggle. My relationship with my husband is more complicated and involves more negotiation (and less fun). I get anxious sometimes thinking about it all. And I wouldn't change any of it. All of the above is true; I'm okay with the ambivalence, and I appreciate it as "normal" and part of this parenting process. We also saw this with my colleague Dr. X, who feels two ways about "working so hard"—on one hand, hard work is consistent with his values and his meaning/purpose, and on the other hand, he wants more time to enjoy life. He's ambivalent.

Bottom line: many choices we make in life have pluses *and* minuses, so ambivalence about change, which comes down to making new choices, is typical, natural, expected, and—thinking back to radical acceptance from the last chapter—something you can embrace, as best you can. I also think about how it's felt to change my eating habits. When I think about what I define as "healthy eating" for myself, I get a little sad. I really love donuts and cupcakes and candy. Sweets are my jam (pun intended). I don't really want to give them up *and* I love how great it feels to be energized and not slogged down (the way I can feel when I'm not making the choices I've decided are best for me in the long run). See? I feel two ways. On one hand I love sweet things *and* on the other hand I love how I feel when I'm making more thoughtful decisions about how much sugar I consume. Both are true.

You'll see I use the word "and" when we talk about the aspects of change we might be ambivalent about, and not "but"; it's intentional. The trick in this behavior change process is to notice the ambivalence and work toward shifting our awareness toward change that matters to us—being aware of what we're excited about and what we're ambivalent about, and being willing to deal with that, rather than avoiding it or behaving as though ambivalence shouldn't or won't exist; it definitely will.

At the same time, ambivalence can leave some of us feeling stuck between a rock and a hard place. When we're thinking about making a behavior change, often some good things and some not so good things keep us stuck. This reality needs all our awareness and attention—you'll need to bring to light potential barriers to change, like your thoughts and behaviors, in order to work with them so they don't stand in your way. And some self-compassion, because it's a human experience like any other; you're not alone or at fault if you're ambivalent. If you can observe ambivalence with what we call your Wise Mind, you can find ways to move forward.

EXERCISE: Your Wise Mind

Who doesn't love a good Venn diagram? (I warned you early on that I'm a bit nerdy.) Here in your hands is possibly the most well-known Venn diagram in the therapy world. Wise Mind is an important concept and one to start playing around with in relation to your ambivalence. Let's first take a look at what Wise Mind is...

WISE MIND

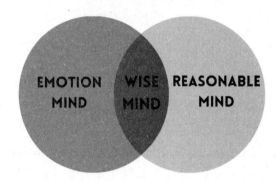

Wise Mind comes from dialectical behavior therapy (DBT), first introduced by Dr. Marsha Linehan, a psychologist and researcher (Linehan 2014). As you can see in the diagram, it is the intersection of Emotion Mind and Reasonable Mind. Think of Emotion Mind as the visceral, uninhibited side of your mind. It's not always bad. This can be joy, excitement, anger, resentment, all of it. When you are in Emotion Mind, you aren't thinking about consequences a ton; you are *feeling*. Reasonable Mind is the data-driven side of your mind, the numbers and sense side. Facts are of top importance when you are in Reasonable Mind; you aren't connected with how you feel. Wise Mind is the state of mind in which our capacities for logic and reason and our emotions come together, and we take into account both our Emotion Mind's and our Reasonable Mind's perspectives. Here is the important part and why I am introducing it to you: being in Wise Mind allows us to act with **wisdom**, **clarity**, and **self-awareness**. We are balanced, thoughtful, and connected with what is important to us—"I know this (Reasonable Mind) and I feel this (Emotion Mind), so I will do this Wise Mindedly."

Here is a simple example. Imagine you are looking for a new vehicle. You go car shopping and are fully enamored with the cherry-apple-red two-seater convertible. It *speaks* to you. That is Emotion Mind showing up, ignoring its high price tag and impracticality for your family. Reasonable Mind, on the other hand, has you drawn to some of the practicalities: a budget friendly, efficient sedan that has great safety features. The sedan doesn't excite you, though. If we let Emotion Mind pick, you would drive home in a convertible that doesn't work for your family of four. If we let Reasonable Mind pick, you would be bored and unhappy with a blasé car that didn't excite you. Wise Mind would help you find a car that speaks to both your emotions and your reasons—one that finds an overlap. Maybe it's a safe coupe in a fun color with cool tech features, or maybe it has one of those giant moon roofs that's convertible-esque and can fit your family in a safe way. Wise Mind is that intersection between what you feel and what you know. Being aware of which state of mind is at play is an important first step; it will help you know if you're leaning in one direction or another and facilitate your ability to access Wise Mind.

Take a moment and think through a change you're considering making. At this point, you likely have an array of changes cropping up in your head. Pick one and see what your Reasonable Mind says about it. What data or facts support your change? Or, what data or facts are there against your change?

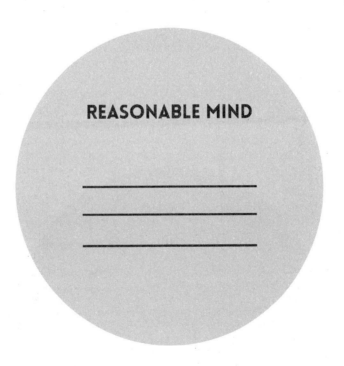

Now, what does Emotion Mind say about the change? How do you *feel* viscerally about it? What feelings show up for you when considering staying the same, and what ones show up when thinking about making the change?

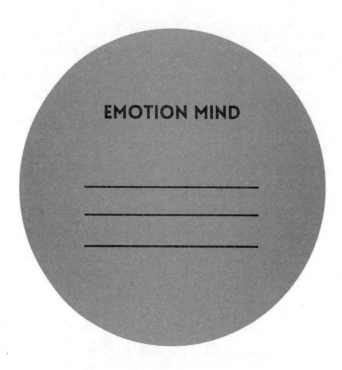

And finally, Wise Mind. How do you feel and what do you know, and where is the intersection?

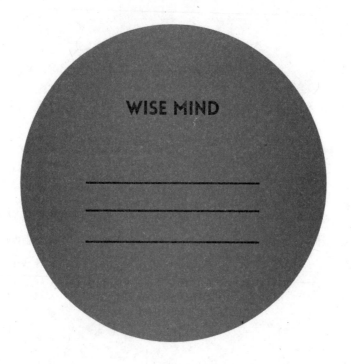

Consider using the Venn diagram and capturing some of what you wrote above. Fill in the emotional side, the reasonable side, and then the wise-minded intersection. This visual is often helpful for folks to consolidate their thinking. You can find the Wise Mind diagram at http://www .newharbinger.com/51543.

FIND YOUR WISE MIND

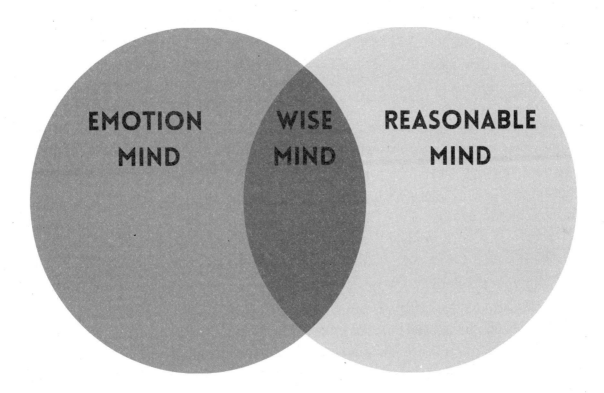

IN YOUR POCKET: Wise Mind is a powerful tool that we will come back to again and again. Keep the Wise Mind Venn diagram close by. You can rip it out from your book (it's your book) or take a pic on your phone. Or, just keep it in your mind's eye. You can also do a web search and quickly find a version of it at any time of the day and night—the internet is a beautiful place sometimes.

Readiness to Change

Now that you've found your Wise Mind, it's time to use it to consider: How ready are you? There is some research that helps identify how ready you are right now (literally in this moment). We can think of it as levels of willingness, often referred to as "stages of change." If you go to http://www.newharbinger.com/51543, you'll find a survey to help you identify which stage of change you fall in right now. And, before you go there, fair warning, your stage of change (i.e., readiness) can change moment to moment. It's what we call a state, so it's going to move around a bit, like a mood—as opposed to a trait, which doesn't change, like your eye color. In fact, it might be helpful to think about your readiness and willingness to change as something that's itself ever changing. That could help you to avoid feeling like you're stuck in one stage or another, or that a particular label in the set of stages perfectly defines you. Right now, we're just getting a snapshot of where you happen to be in this moment. Make sense?

Whether you have taken the assessment or not, here is some info about the stages of change and what they might mean for you:

Precontemplation. These are the folks who aren't thinking about change yet. One of my patients was depressed and used marijuana daily. He was in a bad spot emotionally and couldn't see the connection between his marijuana use and his depression, or the related consequences (missing obligations, for example), so cutting down wasn't even on his radar—it wasn't a change he was considering making.

Odds are if you're reading this book, you won't fall into this category unless someone bought this book for you and is somehow coercing you to read it (it happens!). When you fall into this state of willingness, the best anyone can do is sit beside you and help you see how your behaviors align (or don't align) with your values and goals, so you can figure out if something could or should change, and how. Sometimes we don't know what we don't know or aren't in a place where we can truly see how our behavior is connected to our wellbeing. If this is you or has been you, we got you! And, I don't judge. We've all been there. Remember, "change is hard!"

Contemplation. Our contemplation friends are starting to think about making a change. They have one foot in and one foot out. They're figuring it out and haven't quite committed just yet; they might be feeling stuck. If this is where you fall, show yourself lots of compassion—this is a tough place to be. In fact, a patient once identified this as the toughest place to be. You already know the complex word we use to describe this, "ambivalence": you feel "two ways" about change. It's like you're in a constant battle with yourself. If you're in this stage, we'll work together to figure out which side of the fence you *really* want to sit on.

Preparation. If you're in preparation, you are getting ready to make a positive change. You've thought through whatever change you hope to make; you are weighing the pros and cons of different plans to make it. You are "in it" and ready for what is on the horizon. Chapter 6 will likely help you a ton!

Action. If this is you, bravo! If you're in the action stage, you're doing it. Look at you—making it happen! And, you might not feel completely stable in the change you're making. Remember, change is a process, and you are always testing and learning about your new behaviors. So, in this stage, you might be learning how to manage without your old behaviors. New behaviors almost always mean giving something up—whoomp whoomp—and even when the old behaviors were unhelpful, we can miss them; they were normal for us once.

Recurrence. Who hasn't been there? After working hard at changing a behavior, you have slipped backward. NBD (no big deal)—if or when you end up here, the strategies you learn in this book will help you reconnect with your "why" and get back on the change wagon. The key thing to know is that this is totally normal. In fact, early in my career, a savvy clinician taught me the value of slips and recurrence of old behaviors—these are opportunities to learn! Yup. There is no "failure" in the change process, just opportunities to tap back into our values and rejigger our plans a smidge.

Maintenance. In this stage, you're working to keep up the hard work you started. As you go farther along, you may need to re-evaluate your change strategy. What worked initially might be a bit dated for your current situation, or you might have burned out on how you were doing things. In MI, and in behavior change generally, we're all about the test and learn approach. And even if you're kicking butt in maintenance, you still might need to reassess every now and again. Which is to say, change is hard, and keeping what you've changed intact is hard, too—and not impossible. We will talk more about all of this in chapter 7.

Moving Forward

Here's a recap of what we learned and did in this chapter.

- Identified our buckets or neighborhoods of change so we don't meander aimlessly

- Connected with our Change Master of the Past to connect with the skills and tools we already have onboard (and might have forgotten about)

- Learned an important word—"ambivalence"—and what it means for our change journey

- Found our Wise Mind (and put it in our pocket), another tool to help ground us and help manage the integration of our emotions with facts and data

- Assessed how ready or willing we are for change, or what stage of change we are in right now (in this very moment)

- What else? What are you taking away from this chapter? Take some notes about what stuck with you.

_____

_____

_____

In the next chapter, you'll continue with the MI task known as focusing. We'll look again at the broad directions for change that have taken shape so far and pick out one step we really want to start with. Ready?!

CHAPTER 3

Finding Your Target: Go Easy

A goal properly set is halfway reached.

—Zig Ziglar

Again, think about that wall with dartboards we talked about in the introduction. Each has its own target/bullseye. If you picked up a dart to throw, you wouldn't know which target you were trying to hit, would you? Your thoughts and efforts would be diffused across the dartboards. And imagine if you were trying to hit all the bullseyes at once. Woah! That would be exhausting, and you might just give up. We need to work together to figure out where to start, what our first destination is, so you can hit *that* target first. Then, we can go back and choose another and another because you will now have the skills for whatever journey you might take. That's why the "goal" part of the MI journey is critical—it teaches you how to focus, narrow in on what you can achieve, and achieve it, so you're motivated to keep going.

In this part of our journey, we'll start drilling down on which specific changes you want to make and where it makes the most sense to start. Like everything in this book, this is your journey, and you can choose which exercises make the most sense to you. That said, even if you think you know where you want to focus, consider moving through the exercises and see if they align with your initial thinking. Sometimes we surprise ourselves. And you're here wanting to make a change, so it might be worth a shot to dig a bit deeper into that change, right?

EXERCISE: Focusing

In this exercise, you'll lay all your cards on the table—all the potential directions in which your change journey might go—and pick the one that feels like the best place to start. We can do this any way that makes sense to you. We just talked about dartboards and knowing where to point your dart, at which target. Or, we can be very simple and do what we used to refer to as a bubble chart, with a bunch of circles drawn out on a piece of paper, computer, or whiteboard (digital or literal). One patient even did this in the theme of a solar system with "planets" of change in sizes representing the magnitude of how "big" the change felt. Any way you slice it, our job in this exercise is to consider the various potential goals in what you want to work on and figure out the best place to start.

I often sit with patients and help them think through their goals. They can be so excited to get rolling, and we have to be strategic about where we invest our energy and how we prioritize our efforts. If we jump willy-nilly into a change goal, we might miss something important that's in the way and hit a big speed bump and get dismayed. That might happen anyway, and we'll deal with that later in chapter 7, but why not start in a thoughtful, careful way?

Let's get started with getting started! Go back and look at your buckets from chapter 2. We're going to reach into those buckets and start narrowing down the behaviors inside them.

My buckets were Health, Fun, Family, and Work/Career. Those are big (gigantic!) buckets, and it'll be hard to know where to start until they're narrowed down a smidge. Under health, there is both eating what feels healthy to me (which might even be further narrowed down to eating more fruits and veggies or eating less carbs or processed foods) and being active (narrowed down to "getting more steps," getting in workouts, or simply moving more by using my standing desk). Family is a giant bucket, and I get anxious about thinking about how many behaviors are inside— so, so many (spending more time with my husband and daughter, for example, and one-mindedly focusing on them without getting distracted by work or other responsibilities). As for fun—huh? What's fun? I almost feel like I lost sight of that bucket and need to do some brainstorming there (I used to be/have fun, right?). Again, that's what this exercise is all about—it's hard to know where to start until you narrow your options down, and it's hard to do *that* unless you know what they are.

So, take a moment and capture what behaviors bubble up out of your buckets. If one of your buckets is School, you might think about what's inside that bucket that you want to drive toward— being more organized, staying on top of your assignments, attending class more? Or if Friends is one of your buckets, maybe you want to keep in touch with them, say yes to social events occasionally, or make a trip to visit someone important to you. And, as you do this, you may find you want to add another bucket. That's great. You're digging deeper into yourself and your change and raising your awareness. No judgment here. Capture what bubbles up.

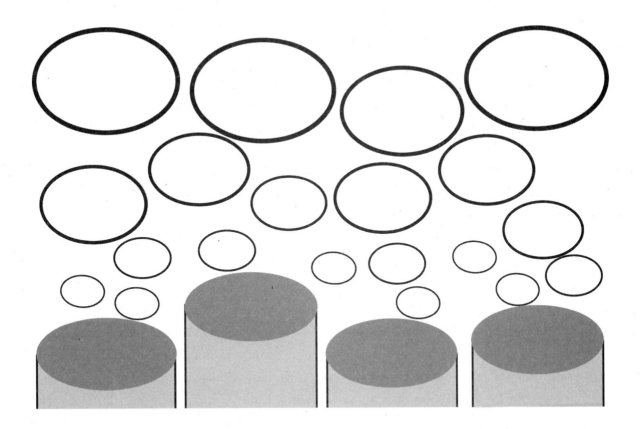

Here, let me remind you of our "test and learn" approach to behavior change. From the various potential opportunities you've brainstormed, you're going to pick an initial starting point (or points)—a specific behavior you think you want to target—and then you can shift and pivot as you start implementing your new behavior and learn what works and what doesn't. Ready? Let's do this.

Step 1: Look at your bubbles, or target behaviors you want to change. Which of those is getting in the way of your living your best life? Which seems to get in the way of your living out your values? What feels like something that comes up often for you? Where does it *feel* like you want to start? I might start, for example, in the Family neighborhood—spending more mindful and present time with my family more often. It's really important to me—one of my top values—and I notice that I'm not living into it regularly. I regularly feel the struggle and I see the opportunity to change there. That is, I see clear ways that making a change would help me to better live out this value (at least I think I do right now).

People I work with are all over the place with these changes. You know why? Ambivalence about changing is normal *and* we're all different in terms of what we might want to change and when we might want to do so. Some want to work on drinking or smoking less, or being more productive, and others want to work on their relationships or curb their spending (and occasionally the two are related). They get to decide how we might work together and figure out where to begin. You are in charge of this. We're partners. That's how we work together. Sometimes people don't feel ready to conquer a change that has been nagging them for a long time, so they start somewhere else that feels more manageable. It's their choice. They know themselves well, just as you know yourself well.

Think about why you picked up this book and why you've made it to this point in the journey—what is driving you. Then think about what's most important, or what feels most accessible to you in this moment; what you really want to start with.

Where will you begin?

My starting target: _____

Step 2: Let's give that starting target some "oomph." Pause and notice how this starting point aligns with your values. Which values is the goal consistent with? For me, the Family bucket is right up there at the top of my values (Loved, Loving, Family). Look back at your values from chapter 2 and note some core values that are relevant here.

Values alignment: _____

_____

_____

Step 3: Come up with an un-SMART goal. You may be familiar with SMART (Specific, Measurable, Achievable, Relevant, Timely) goals from your place of work or previous therapy. I confess I am not the biggest fan. It's a great framework in some instances—and it can be limiting and somewhat demoralizing at times; it can put us in a tiny corner. At the same time, it helps to have a goal be defined and actionable so we know when we're hitting the target; if a goal is too vague, you can't give yourself credit for it. That is, if you just say, "work out more," how do you know what "more" is and whether you're hitting that target? If instead, you say, "work out three to four times a week," it gives you something specific to strive for. Conversely, though, if you want to start meditating regularly, for instance, "daily-ish," as opposed to "daily," is a helpful goal. It gives you some space for the inevitable days you won't quite be able to keep your commitment, and builds in some compassion for those times, which will serve you well. We don't need to be overcontrolled perfectionists here, at the start of the change process. That will demoralize us and we will lose this war with our inner critic.

We need a sweet spot. So, let's get a little clarity on your goal so you can answer yes or no when asked, "Have you done the thing or not?" (Have you worked out? Have you checked and taken action on all your emails before logging off for the day? Have you started a conversation with a new person this week? Did you go to bed at a reasonable time? Yes or no? This will make your progress easy to monitor and track.) Now draft your goal in a way we can ask the yes/no question. Mine might say "Having dinner at home with the family a couple nights a week." It's not perfect *and* it's a start. One patient's simple goal was something like "Drinking alcohol just two to three days a week and no more than two to three drinks each time." Another's was "Get to bed by 10 p.m.; stop using devices about an hour before." Another patient: "Save 10 percent of every paycheck for a housing down payment."

What's a simple goal you can start with? What will be your first step?

Simple Goal: _____

> **IN YOUR POCKET:** Now that you've got this simple goal down, how can you find ways to keep yourself mindful of it? You might jot it down on a notecard or set up a recurring alert, as a way to keep the goal "in your pocket" and top of mind. This is where you are starting. You could take a pic of something related to the goal that will trigger an association for you. For instance, I might change my phone's home screen to a picture of my family to remind myself of my goal of connecting with them. In the sections to come, we'll talk more about tracking and monitoring your "progress" toward this goal—and just having a reminder near you is a great place to begin. It's easy to forget even when you feel so motivated right now. So take a moment and think through a way to remind yourself.

Now, if you were successful, you've got a clear, valued, and actionable first goal down—a place to start. Good job sticking with this journey. This is important to you and you are working hard at it. Even if you haven't quite yet been successful in narrowing it down, you are reading these words and are still engaged in the process. That is something and this all matters. You can come back to this focusing task again and again.

Now let's start talking about how to help you achieve that goal. Change is hard, yes, and very possible. Let's turn to another tool we'll be using throughout this book to keep ourselves on track and engaged with change: mindful awareness.

Building Your Awareness Muscle

You might be wondering what this mindful awareness stuff is doing in a book about behavior change. Mindful awareness as we will use it here might not be exactly what you're thinking. Unless it's your thing, we're not going to get all squishy and "Zen Buddha" here. And, we are going to use mindful awareness to help you in a bunch of different ways. Before we talk about the application, let's define mindfulness: "Mindfulness is awareness that arises through paying attention, on purpose, in the present moment, non-judgmentally…in the service of self-understanding and wisdom," says mindful guru Jon Kabat-Zinn (mindful.org 2022).

Being aware of ourselves and our behaviors is key to understanding what we are doing and how we are doing it. Do you know how much happens outside our awareness? Think about it for a moment. What are you doing right now? Presumably breathing—although I often notice I've been holding my breath when I'm thinking or concentrating intently or when I'm anxious about something—and for the most part breathing happens without awareness. Similarly, many habits (unhelpful or helpful ones) happen automatically without us being aware of them, like nail biting, hair twirling, cracking your knuckles, or other nervous habits. Ultimately, mindfulness will help you be more aware of what you are or are not doing. Awareness is a powerful tool, both in general and when you want to make, and stick to, a change in your thinking or your behavior. Using your mindfulness muscle is going to help a ton with that. Let's see what that's like.

EXERCISE: Beginner's Mind

There are many different ways to approach and learn mindfulness. One of my favorites leans into something we refer to as "beginner's mind" (Suzuki 2020). This is often how I introduce the concept of nonjudgmental awareness with patients. Before I describe it in too much detail, let's just do it! If you are willing, follow me…

Locate something that you can eat. Anything: fruit, gum, pretzel, chocolate, whatever is available. Try not to be too picky; just grab *some*thing. It's important to notice your judgments even at this point. For example, I usually do this exercise with raisins—and I never knew people had such strong feelings and thoughts about shriveled up grapes!

Okay, take whatever food you grabbed and place the object in the palm of your hand. Look at it as if you have never seen it before. Seriously, pretend you have dropped down from outer space and have never seen this object before. Get curious.

Allow your eyes to scan every part of it. Look at it and *really* notice it. Move it around. Observe where it's hard and where it's soft. Become aware of where the light shines on it and where there are shadows. Look at the colors.

And, while you are doing this, observe any thoughts you might be having, including judgments—judgments about the object, the activity, or me and this book—notice any thoughts that show up. What is your mind saying to yourself? Then bring your attention back to the object. Observe it as if you have never seen it before.

Now, with the object in the palm of your hand, look at it again from different angles. Poke it a bit. Roll it around. Maybe even squeeze it between your fingers. What does it feel like? Does it make a sound? How heavy or light is it? Remember, you've just dropped in and have never seen this before. You are curious and collecting data about this object.

Now bring it up to your nose. Breathe in. Smell it. What does it smell like? And notice how your mind and body so easily knew how to work together to "bring it up to your nose." It probably happened automatically—bring awareness to even some of those automatic behaviors.

Where is your mind at? What thoughts are you noticing? If your mind is saying something like *What kind of exercise am I doing?!* or *I must not be doing this right*, just notice those thoughts and then bring your mind back to the object. Over and over, no matter what thoughts or emotions might arise, bring your mind back to the object.

Now bring the object up to your lips. Again, notice how your mind can move your body naturally, without your explicit command. Notice even how your mouth might get "ready" to receive the object. It happens. Heck, your mouth might even start watering during this exercise. Whatever might happen, just notice that.

Take the object into your mouth and notice any urge you might have to bite down. Move it around in your mouth. Play with it a bit, moving it from side to side. And then, when you're ready, very mindfully and with your full awareness, take a bite. As you do, feel your teeth and your tongue work together to chew. Notice the smells, the tastes, the textures. Be aware of all of it and be aware of your thoughts and judgments around it.

Finally, when you're ready, swallow, with full awareness. Follow the object down to your stomach and observe that your body is now one object heavier.

Take a moment and sit back and think about what you learned from this exercise. What did you learn about your mind and your attention? How easy or hard was this?

_____

_____

_____

Now, consider how you could apply it in this behavior change journey. How might a beginner's mind approach to your behavior journey be helpful? What role will mindful awareness play as you work to change a behavior that's important to you? Capture some of those observations here.

_____

_____

_____

Many people are surprised by how "mindless" they often are in their life. So much of what we do happens automatically, and that's part of what makes behavior change so hard. We have deeply worn-in behavior pathways that we get drawn back to over and over. Mindfulness is a muscle you can grow and flex to help you be more aware of when you are and aren't acting in line with your goals and values.

Of course, keeping your mind trained on one thing at a time is a tough skill to develop and master. Odds are the Beginner's Mind exercise might have been tough for you. Even the mindfulness gurus struggle with it sometimes. Ultimately, the awareness of the struggle is part of the journey; it's a sign you're being mindful of what's coming up for you. So try not to judge yourself—remembering the "nonjudgmentally" part of the definition—or get discouraged. Mindfulness is a practice, which means you need to do it often. You'll find it's a lot like strengthening a muscle; do it over and over again and you'll make progress. Go slow and steady with lots of self-compassion along the way.

If an exercise to access beginner's mind isn't your jam, there are plenty of other opportunities to practice mindfulness and awareness. Another favorite exercise I do with patients is called "leaves on a stream," where you visualize a flowing stream in your mind—one with leaves floating along the top. You take each thought, feeling, or sensation that enters your awareness and place it on a leaf so you can watch it float by. You do this for a few minutes, noticing how fast or slow the stream flows, letting the thoughts, feelings, and sensations you've placed on the leaves make their way through your mind. And you notice when you get distracted, which again is not just typical but expected. Ultimately, "leaves on a stream" is a way to notice your thoughts and see them as separate from you—create some distance from the thoughts in your brain and from yourself. In cognitive behavioral therapy (CBT), we have a mantra: "Just because you think it, doesn't make it true"; this exercise reflects that. And you don't have to stick with the leaves metaphor; you can do this exercise with thoughts on clouds in the sky or as pieces of luggage circling a luggage carousel, whatever visualization you like. There are also several apps and opportunities online to practice what's known as "formal" mindfulness—exercises like these that you do as a dedicated, sit-down practice for a certain length of time. What used to be reserved for "serious meditators" is now available to all of us to improve our awareness and attention.

There's also what's called informal mindfulness practice, which is the practice of using mindful attention in our day-to-day life experiences. You can use your awareness muscle in so many ways throughout the day: brush your teeth mindfully (one tiny stroke at a time), walk mindfully (notice how your legs move), look at each letter in each word you are reading mindfully, find your feet (you know that one already!); the list goes on and on.

Let's look at how this all comes together for someone trying to make important changes in their life. A patient of mine had been thinking about stopping nicotine use for, well, forever. Many had implored her to stop since she started in her teens—her parents, her friends, her romantic partners. And yet, she just couldn't shake the habit. At some point she had switched from cigarettes to vaping and found that was "good enough." Then, she had a health scare, while also in a new relationship, and the scales tipped. Having a new, caring partner to support her behavior change while also having more salient reasons (health) made change not just more likely, but also feel more possible. She was ready.

We had already spent time identifying her values (family, autonomy, health, contribution, creativity, love) and the various neighborhoods or buckets of change. She felt she was doing well in her career and with her family and relationships—and, she felt, she really needed to focus on health. The nicotine use had been nagging at her for a long time. She talked about how shameful she felt vaping. She was a professional in a corporate setting who would "sneak off" to vape, and she judged herself every time. It wasn't who she wanted to be. And now that she'd been in urgent care for a health scare, she decided it was time to really make a change in this part of her life. So together we thought through some options for where to start—she could get nicotine patches, gum, or lozenges; or she could get medication from her physician to help; or she could quit cold turkey. The cold turkey plan felt too overwhelming, so she decided to start by reducing her vaping use by making it "less easy"—less of an automatic behavior—to vape. She decided to do that by moving her vape to a high-up shelf so she'd have a harder time accessing it, introducing some friction into what had once been seamless. She wasn't ready to "get rid" of the vape, and this was a move toward her first step, reducing her use. Not a bad place to start!

Tracking Your Progress

One thing we know from research, including my own, is that tracking (aka self-monitoring)—keeping track of what you are doing and when you are doing it—can help you increase awareness of how you are doing with your goals (Michie et al. 2009; Chia, Anderson, and McLean 2019). It gives you data you can consider when it comes to how best to make a change stick—a way to figure out what's easy and what's hard, what's working and what's not.

Self-monitoring is also a space where you can get super sophisticated and complex if you want, or you can be simple and straightforward, or, if you hate this kind of thing, you can skip it altogether, because this is your journey and you're doing this your way. Still, if you want my advice, I'm glad to step up here and say this often is one of the more helpful pieces of behavior change, one that really makes a difference. So, even if your mind is telling you that you might hate it, it might be worth mindfully acknowledging this judgment—and then giving it a try.

The important thing to remember here is that we're tracking the behavior you are trying to change—not the outcome necessarily. If your goal is to stop vaping, like the patient we discussed above, then you track when you do and don't vape. The "feeling good" part might come later, and the health benefits much later—or maybe never because what you're actually doing is preventing certain health outcomes rather than working toward them. Similarly, if you're working on flossing more, you track which days you flossed; it's not as important if you have reduced your cavities yet or not. Focus on your simple goal and the yes or no question you used to structure it, and you can start as simply as tracking yes or no.

On the next page is a simple chart you can use to track your progress keeping up with your goal. There's also space to reflect on and jot down what worked and what still needs work at the end of each week. (You can also download more copies of this chart at http://www.newharbinger .com/51543.) Another option is to make notes in your calendar—paper or electronic, whatever you use—or use some other strategy to track. Some people even like to take pics of their progress, like grabbing a selfie of you out on a walk or snapping a pic of your latest healthy meal. (Also, sharing that picture in a group chat or posting it online somewhere might be another helpful way to keep yourself on track while involving a supportive community who can rally around you.) There are tons of apps you can download, too, if you are techy and love data. You can also do all of the above. This is your journey.

SIMPLE GOAL TRACKER

SIMPLE GOAL:

WEEK	M	T	W	TH	F	S	SU
	○	○	○	○	○	○	○
	○	○	○	○	○	○	○
	○	○	○	○	○	○	○
	○	○	○	○	○	○	○
	○	○	○	○	○	○	○
	○	○	○	○	○	○	○

WHAT WORKED:

WHAT STILL NEEDS WORK:

If tracking your progress feels like a good approach for you, pick a data-collection strategy that aligns with your personality. Personally, as a researcher, I *love* data, so I have apps on my phone that give me tons of output (sometimes even too much, despite my love of information). I also devote some attention in my tracking to what I'm doing on a daily basis (e.g., what kinds of food I'm eating, how much I'm exercising). I find it helps me understand more of what is going on with my body and make decisions that are more in line with my goals and values, rather than getting sidetracked by sensations or stimuli that I'm just not mindful of. Patients similarly report that this is one of the more helpful tools in their behavior change journey. One patient thought it was the coolest thing to use an app that tracked the amount of time she hadn't been drinking alcohol, which also calculated how much money she was saving. Could be fun, right?

Counting days—the number of days, often in a row, that you have been successful at something you're working on—is a common strategy in the behavior change world, like a "streak" you might see in an app or a digital platform. The one caution with streaks or counting days is this: the "f*ck its" we talked about might show up. Sometimes if you break your streak, your mind gets dismayed and you think *f*ck it* and go off your behavior change journey altogether, minimizing the progress you've made. Here's a piece of advice: if you go the route of counting days or working on a streak, try to keep your focus on the days you *did* the change, not the days you *didn't* do the change, even if you go off path for a day or two. This can help manage or even prevent the f*ck its. You know yourself. Review the options for tracking and think about what would help you most effectively.

Another useful tracking tool is reflection. So consider this: once you've practiced with a chosen strategy for a while (a few days or a few weeks), come back here and note some observations about what the experience was like—what was difficult, what was easy; which skills you might have used (radical acceptance, Wise Mind, mindfulness, monitoring and tracking); how you feel about the progress you've made; and how you feel about your simple goal now that you've had a while to implement it. Pro tip: Set a reminder on your phone or calendar to remember to do this. You may have stopped tracking—because tracking is itself a behavior and, well, behavior change is hard—and this will in itself be a good reminder. Notice: Did anything get easier, or harder? How do you feel about your goal now? Are you still tracking? Why or why not?

_____

_____

_____

_____

The point here is not to criticize yourself, whether you've been successful or not. It's to encourage you to reflect on your efforts at working toward your simple goal and to make a consistent, ongoing practice of considering what's gone well and what might need some fine tuning. This sort of reflection is an awareness-raising exercise, and it can sometimes be helpful in continuing your progress toward a goal and maintaining a goal or behavior change once you've initially achieved it.

Moving Forward

Here's a recap of what we learned and what we did in this chapter:

- Defined our high-level goals

- Narrowed down to a simple goal

- Flexed our awareness muscle

- Learned about beginner's mind

- Explored the value and some methods of self-monitoring/tracking

- What else are you taking away from this chapter? What stuck with you?

_____

_____

_____

The next chapter kicks off part 3 of the book, "Evoking," where we really start to dig out your reasons for change and consolidate more of your motivation. Chapter 4 will get you listening to the active ingredient in MI: "change talk," or the ways we talk to ourselves and others about change. It's a big, exciting chapter, so get ready.

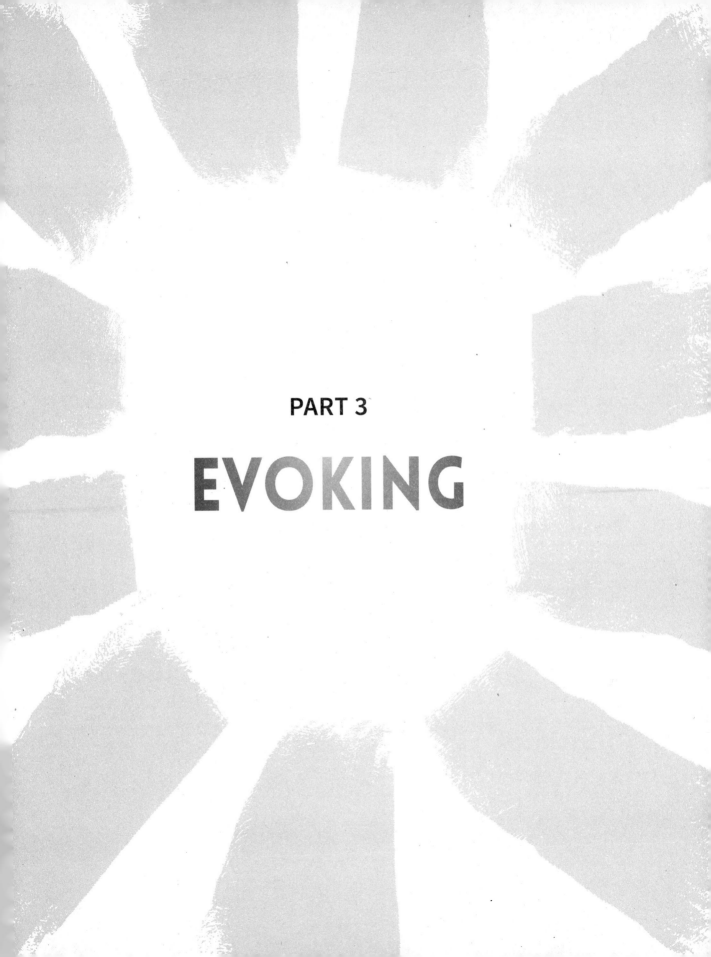

PART 3

EVOKING

CHAPTER 4

Learning Change Talk

People are the undisputed experts on themselves. No one has been with them longer, or knows them better than they do themselves.

—Bill Miller and Steve Rollnick, founders of Motivational Interviewing

We've come so far. Now it's time to dive into the nitty gritty—the behavior science that will help you start the change process and stick with it; what, in MI, is considered the really important stuff, the active ingredient in the whole approach. We often think about behavior change in terms of what we covered in the last chapter—setting actionable goals, tracking our progress toward those goals, and working our way, small goal by small goal, up to achieving our high-level valued directions in life.

What makes MI effective—and distinctive—is how it encourages us to pay attention to the secret ingredient that we *don't* often think about, which is how you talk to both yourself and others about change. We're often drawn to jump right into how to change without pausing to consider why we want this change. We call this talk about change "change talk" (genius, right?) (Miller and Rollnick 2012). We researchers know that calling forth talk about *why* you might want to change and encouraging that kind of talk can create hope. We also know that certain kinds of talk are more likely to leave you feeling discouraged and demotivated. So in this chapter we're going to think about how you can become more aware of the aspects of your change process that will help you change. We'll consider the type and strength of language you're using both inside your head and with others, which helps us peek into your motivation. Finally, you'll look at your own change talk and how to leverage it most effectively as you continue to progress through simple goals and toward bigger ones.

Types of Change Talk

Change talk comes in two main flavors: preparatory and mobilizing. Preparatory change talk is the "getting ready" change talk, the things you say when you're thinking about change, assessing your ability and interest in changing, and preparing for change. Mobilizing change talk refers to the things you say when you're getting ready to change or are already rallying to do it. We have an acronym for the different types of change talk you might utter across the span of getting ready and just thinking about why you might want to change to being in action: DARN-CAT (sorry to all you cat lovers out there!).

D-desire: "I want to do this."

A-ability: "I can do this." or "I have done this in the past."

R-reasons: "I will do this because…" or "If I do this it will change my life in these ways…"

N-need: "I *need* to do this or else…" or "My doctor tells me I need to do this" or "I have to make this change."

C-commitment: "I am going to do this."

A-action: "I started working on this behavior change by…"

T-taking steps: "I started doing part of this by…" or "I made a step toward doing this by…" or "I scheduled an appointment for…"

DARN-CAT is an important tool to identify and possibly even stimulate change talk (e.g., thinking about change, communicating change).

Have you already started to think about and notice your own DARN-CATs? It's been shown that the more change talk someone uses, the more likely they are to make and stick with a change (Moyers et al. 2007). That seems like a "no duh" research finding, yet it's still super powerful. It's easy for us to become bogged down with the anti-change side of our arguments, the voice of doubt and resistance, like *Giving up substances is hard, it's scary; if I do it, I won't have any friends because they all use.* We could instead help ourselves build a big pile of DARN-CATs! Knowing that we can do things to help increase change talk and motivation—and vice versa—is a really powerful tool. Strategies to intervene in and change a client's change talk are skillful and meaningful ones that highly trained clinicians leverage in treatment, to results that sometimes feel magical, even, to clients they serve. Fun fact: change talk used to be called "self-motivational statements," and knowing how to elicit and reinforce change talk from *yourself* is going to help with your motivation. I am here to help you figure out how to do some of this for yourself.

Let's bring this to life a little bit more. Think about your simple goal from last chapter, or a general change in one of your buckets that you have been contemplating, and see where you are with your DARN-CATs. (You can also download this worksheet at http://www.newharbinger.com/51543 to make copies.)

DARN-CATS WORKSHEET

Simple Goal: _____

D-desire: Why do you want to make this change? _____

_____

A-ability: What have you done like this before? What tools do you have onboard to help? What about you as a person would make this possible? _____

_____

R-reasons: What are some reasons you might want to make this change? _____

_____

N-need: Why do you need to make this change? What makes it important to you? _____

_____

C-commitment: How committed are you to making this change? _____

_____

A-action: What actions are you doing to make this change? What are you ready, willing, or preparing to do? _____

_____

T-taking steps: What steps have you already taken toward the change? _____

_____

Wait… Did you capture reading this book in your change talk above? You are reading these words, holding this book, giving it at least some of your attention. That is action for sure. You will also notice that sometimes in the change journey you don't give yourself credit for the steps you are taking. Try to use your nonjudgmental awareness muscle to take in the whole field of DARN-CATs—the big and small parts of change.

You also might have noticed, as you were thinking or writing, that the opposite of change talk was coming up—that is, language that supports sustaining your current behaviors, the status quo, your baseline; what we call "sustain talk." Basically, anytime you catch yourself thinking or talking about staying the same, you are using sustain talk. And, sorry to break it to you, but the more you talk about staying the same, guess what? The more likely you are to *not* change. This is a meaningful point, so start to listen to yourself and be aware of where you are in your change journey. Remember stages of change from chapter 2? This is all related.

YES, BUT…

When you were thinking about your DARN-CATs, you might have heard a little voice in your head saying, *Yes, but…* and felt drawn to qualify. *I really want to stop drinking, but I haven't been able to do it before.* Or, *My doctor says I need to watch my sugars, but I have a sweet tooth.* Or, *I want to get healthier, but I have failed so many times before.* Or, *I really want to write that novel/run that marathon/pursue my true calling, but I am not a disciplined enough person to succeed.*

It can help to be mindful of the "Yes, but's." This is a tough one. We often catch ourselves saying or thinking, *Yes, but…* I sometimes watch a patient's face and as I notice their brow furrow, I'll ask, "What is the 'Yes, but' in your head?" We are so great about giving some change talk and then snatching it back or dampening it with some sustain talk after the "but." "I really want to work out regularly, but I am so busy." "I need to start flossing, but I keep forgetting." "I started reducing my drinking, but just can't stick with it."

Quick piece of advice to take or leave. First, flip the script, literally: start with sustain talk and next change "but" to "and" so you get "I am so busy *and* I really want to work out regularly." Or, like my vaping patient, "I am so used to vaping and it's not consistent with who I want to be." A small shift in our language and our thinking can lead to a change in our behavior (and vice-versa, for the record; a shift in our behavior leads to changes in our thinking). This may seem like a nuanced point—and I wouldn't spend precious real estate in this book or our lives if it wasn't meaningful.

EXERCISE: Looking at Your Change Talk

Okay! Let's test out some of what we learned above. You may be thinking, *I wonder how this change talk business applies to me...* (*And, how do I apply Jedi mind tricks to myself?!*) Hang tight; we'll get there. One way we bring this to life for patients is with rulers. Let's try this together now, if you are up for it. Refer back to your simple goal from chapter 3 if you jotted one down.

What change are you working on making *right now*?

_____

Importance Ruler

1. On a scale from 0 to 10, where 0 is "not at all important" and 10 is "completely important," how important would you say making this change is to you?

_____

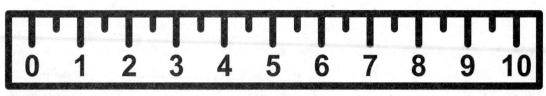

NOT AT ALL   NEUTRAL   COMPLETELY
IMPORTANT   IMPORTANT

2. Now, muse on this question: Why are you at a _____ (number you selected above) and not a 0? Why did you choose that number? Pro tip: If answering this feels funky to you, try talking out loud and recording yourself, and then taking notes from that recording.

_____

_____

_____

_____

3. Notice what you captured above, and apply DARN-CAT to it. What parts of what you said fell into the Desire, Ability, Reasons, or Need categories? What are you already doing

toward making that change (the CAT part of DARN-CAT)? Look for and listen for change talk. What did you discover?

_____

_____

_____

_____

When we ask how "important," we are really asking how motivated you are. So look again at your answers above and let that sink in…

Confidence Ruler

This is related but different, so consider giving it a go….

1. On a scale from 0 to 10, where 0 is "not at all confident" and 10 is "completely confident," how confident are you that you can make this change in, say, the next couple of weeks?

_____

```
| 0  1  2  3  4  5  6  7  8  9  10 |
```

NOT AT ALL   NEUTRAL   COMPLETELY
CONFIDENT   CONFIDENT

2. Now, write down your answer to this question: Why are you at a _____ (number you selected above) and not a 0? Why did you choose that number? Again, try recording yourself talking out loud and then taking notes from that recording if that's helpful to you.

_____

_____

_____

_____

Let's look at what you captured here and apply DARN-CAT to it. Which parts of what you said fell into the Commitment, Action, or Taking steps change talk versus Desire, Ability, Reasons, and Need? Look for and listen for change talk. What are you noticing?

_____

_____

_____

_____

Think of your confidence rating as how ready you feel. And "readiness" isn't just personal; it's also environmental—about the resources you might or might not have. Think back to the COM-B (Capability + Opportunity + Motivation = Behavior change) model of change. Do you have the tools to launch into this change? Do you need some additional skills? Also, what's the size or scale of the change—how important is it in the grand scheme of your life? How aligned is this change to your values? That, too, can influence our readiness and confidence profoundly. Something can be super important (10 out of 10) and you don't feel confident at all that you can do it (2 or 3), maybe even *because* it's so important. That is much different from someone who feels uber confident (10 out of 10) that they can make a given change but just doesn't see it as important (1 or 2). I sometimes hear people who smoke in this latter group: "I can totally quit smoking today. It's easy. I just don't want to." This is a motivational challenge more than a skills challenge and requires a different approach. And there are some people who smoke, like the patient I told you about who vaped, who aren't very confident at all (4 or 5), and to whom quitting is very important (8 or 9). In that case, they need tactical help and assistance with skills and a plan.

How Strong Are Your DARN-CATs?

Based on the research, more important than figuring out where your change talk falls in the DARN-CAT is getting a sense of the quantity and quality (strength) of change talk to indicate where you are on the change journey. One of the easiest ways to bring the value and importance of the strength of change talk to life is with some simple examples. First, whether you are married or not, you're likely familiar with the standard marriage vows used in typical American culture. So, imagine a couple is engaged and standing at the altar, getting ready to commit to marriage for the rest of their lives. The wedding officiant turns to one of the betrothed and says something like "Do you take this person to be your wife, to live together in (holy) matrimony, to love her, to honor her, to comfort her, and to keep her in sickness and in health, forsaking all others, for as long as you both shall live?" and the answer is…"I *think* I can" or "I *hope* so" or "I will work on it" or even "I want to but I'm not sure." That would cause quite a stir, huh? I would have run from my husband citing lack of strong change talk! The stereotypical, committed answer we are looking for is an affirmative, unwavering "I do."

Similarly, imagine you're in a court of law and are about to testify. The judge turns to you and asks, "Do you swear to tell the truth, the whole truth, and nothing but the truth?" and you answer, "I'm not sure" or "I will try" or "I'm working on that." You would not be allowed to testify. The judge wants a clear, committed answer like "I do" or "I will." No wishy-washiness; people don't trust that level of commitment. So, just as we care about the quantity of change talk, it's also very meaningful to listen for the quality and strength of change talk. If I hear a patient saying something like "I'm not sure" or "I will try…?" (question mark intentional), I know we have some work to do together on level of commitment and motivation—just like we're doing here. If you are noticing you are wishy-washy, pat yourself on the back for mindfully noticing—and know that we also need to find ways to shore that motivation up!

So as you dig around and pull out your own change talk, take note of the amount *and* the strength of it. Do so mindfully, knowing that it helps to understand where you are on this journey, and that if your change talk just doesn't feel strong or meaningful enough for you to feel ready to take on the change, we can work to strengthen it or draw it out.

EXERCISE: Flexing Your Change Talk Muscles

Remember, the more you talk about changing, the more likely you are to change. I often elicit change talk from patients by asking evocative questions about what they want to do, why they want to do it, and how important they feel it is. My MI training tells me that when I do this it helps orient and empower them to feel that change is possible. Let's try a version of this now. I'm going to offer you the opportunity to record yourself answering the following questions aloud, rather than just writing your answers down. So, before you dive in, set up some way to record yourself. You can use an app on your phone (voice memo works), your laptop, or go old school with a voice recorder. This is not a transcription exercise. There is value in literally recording yourself speaking.

Now, find yourself a quiet place to record.

Once you're settled in, think about a change you are considering making. And answer these questions out loud while recording yourself:

1. *What change are you considering making? (Describe the change in detail. What would it look like when you've changed?)*

2. *Why do you want to make this change?*

3. *How could you go about making this change? What would help you be successful?*

4. *Really lean in… What are the three best reasons to make this change?*

5. *Finally, how important is this change to you on a scale from 0 (not at all important) to 10 (couldn't be more important)?*

6. *Why?*

Stop the recording.

Play it back. Listen to yourself talking about change. Yes, I know how hard it is to listen to your own voice, and if this weren't a meaningful exercise, I wouldn't be suggesting it. If it helps, try pretending (or practicing self-compassion!) and remind yourself that you are listening to someone you really care about, love, and want to help.

Now, really listen. We call this "tuning your ear." Capture some notes about the DARN-CATs you heard. Notice any of the "I want to…," "I could…," "I ought to…," "My reasons for doing this are…"—all the language that indicates your motivation for change. What were some of the meaningful change nuggets you collected? What did you hear?

_____

_____

_____

_____

_____

_____

Finally, read back the notes you took on your change reasons out loud. Notice how you're talking yourself into change. Go you!

Now, answer this question (you can do it out loud and record it or just take some notes directly):

Knowing all you know, having listened to your change talk, what do you think you'll do?

_____

_____

_____

_____

This is an important exercise to slow down your thinking process and get to know yourself a bit more. Our minds process so rapidly that we sometimes don't catch everything. The act of talking aloud probably facilitated your hearing yourself and listening to what you are thinking about change more than you had previously.

When I have patients do this activity and listen, *really listen*, to themselves, they're sometimes surprised, delighted, and motivated by what they hear. One patient listened to the recording of himself talking through his desire to change his relationship with his in-laws and heard himself mentioning all the reasons he wanted to make the change (to improve his relationship with his partner; to facilitate his kids' relationships with their grandparents; to get much needed childcare help). He also heard himself starting to think through how he could improve the relationship with his father-in-law in particular: he drew from his knowledge of improving teams at work and remembered the concept of "assuming positive intent," where you come from the stance that someone has good, positive intentions in their behavior even if your Emotion Mind has a knee-jerk reaction to them. Most importantly, he was open to all that he was hearing because *he* was doing the talking and someone wasn't talking at him and telling him what to do. He also realized that he already had lots of what he needed onboard. He just had to leverage it. He walked away from the recording feeling hopeful and more engaged in his own change journey—all because he listened to himself!

IN YOUR POCKET: This is a moment to step back and capture some of your personal change talk. Snap a photo of the reflections you jotted down to keep your DARN-CATs close. Or maybe hang on to that change talk recording so you can play it again; or in time, re-record it as your change journey proceeds. And continue to observe how your DARN-CATs are helping you along your journey.

Stepping into Planning

You flexed your change talk muscle and it's going strong. Now we can start to really think through how to get you mobilized toward making the change happen. Above you answered the question "What do you think you'll do?" In chapter 6, we'll explore planning in more detail. For now, think about one small step in the direction of change you are willing to make. One small yet meaningful move…

_____

_____

_____

_____

EXERCISE: The Miracle/Magic Question

This is a classic exercise that clinicians use to help individuals connect with their internal motivation for change and to draw out some of their change talk by envisioning or imagining that the change has already occurred. So, bear with me as we take a journey into our imagination…

This may seem like an unusual question, and let's try it out and see where it takes us.

Imagine you're living your life as it is, normally—living the "status quo." Then, you head off to bed and fall asleep as usual…

While asleep, something happens—a miracle (or magic or you won the lottery or something bonkers like that). When you awake, the change that you have been considering throughout this whole book is done, completely, perfectly. It's happened! The thing you have been stuck on is accomplished.

As you wake up and realize this has happened, what do you notice in your life? What is different?

_____

_____

_____

_____

How do you move about your life without this behavior change bugging you? What is your life like now that you were magically "changed"?

_____

_____

_____

_____

Now, returning to "real" life in the present… Look back at your answers. Notice how you felt. Use your mindful muscle to think about how this feels in your body and what kinds of thoughts are coming up for you. What would it *feel* like to have made this change?

_____

_____

_____

_____

This tool can help you connect with your values, elicit your change talk, and give you an important perspective. I use a version of this with myself often... I fast-forward my life in my head and picture myself as an older woman in my last phase of life (aged eighties+). I am happy and healthy enjoying life and I look back on this moment in my story—on myself as a woman in her forties writing a book on behavior change. The older, wiser version of myself often giggles at my current self, thinking of how this moment in time *feels* so big and meaningful, and in the grand scheme of my life, this is just a moment. I then ask her advice on how to get through this moment, and she is a wise, sassy older lady who helps me hear what I need to move forward, one tiny step at a time: "Find your feet."

Moving Forward

Again, here's a recap of what we learned and did in this chapter.

- Learned to distinguish change talk from sustain talk and covered how more change talk = more change

- Reviewed a nifty acronym for identifying change talk: DARN-CAT

- Assessed our readiness to change using the Importance and Confidence Rulers

- Did a visioning exercise—the Miracle/Magic Question—to help draw out change talk and think about what your life will be like when you have made the change you are planning

- What else are you taking away from this chapter? What stuck with you?

_____

_____

_____

In the next chapter, we will spend time reviewing how to draw out and reinforce change talk in ourselves using MI communication skills—and we'll learn how you can leverage those skills to communicate with others more effectively. It's a handy chapter for this stage in your change journey!

CHAPTER 5

Communicate Your Positive Change

We have two ears and one mouth so that we can listen twice as much as we speak.

—Epictetus

This week I restarted a Couch to 5K program again. I had been wanting to do it, had been thinking about doing it, and knew I could do it since I have completed it a few times in the past. That's a lot of change talk—all of it happening in my head, of course. What was it that ultimately got me moving into action? It was the act of communicating my change and mobilizing others around me so that they understood what I was up to and could help me with my change. I talked about it. I texted about it. I wrote on social media about it. I gave myself a pep talk by reflecting my DARN-CATs, like we learned in chapter 4. And I asked for help from people around me—not just to keep me accountable ("How did your Couch to 5K workout go?"), but also to facilitate my ability to do the thing, to get out and "run," because I knew there were people in my life excited to see me progress and succeed. Those people could also help create the time and space for me to run—my husband might make sure my daughter got off to school while I was running, or someone at work could handle something for me so I would have extra time to go for a run, for example.

When we're engaged in the project of creating the lives we want, having the support of others around us, both practical and emotional, is invaluable. And it's also key to notice what I did *not* do while I worked to secure that support for myself. I didn't yell or demand help. When I asked for help, I explained myself and was kind, caring, and compassionate to myself and others in that process. And now, I am doing the thing I set out to do. (Week 1 in the books!) Look at me go!

Even though I am the one making the moves throughout my tiny town, I'm not really doing it alone. I need help and to get that help, I need to know how to talk to others—and how to listen to myself. Think back to the COM-B model (Capability + Opportunity + Motivation = Behavior change) and how all components can involve other people. I may need someone to help me with the actual tasks involved in my behavior change, like a teacher or a coach (capability), or I might need another person to help create the time and space for me to do the new behavior (opportunity), or I might need someone in my corner, cheering me on in a very compassionate, empathic, supportive way (motivation). Communicating with ourselves and others is a meaningful part of our change journey.

As we learned in the last chapter, motivation involves how I talk to myself—what I'm saying and how strong that language is. If you're able to have good supportive communication with yourself and to evoke motivation and reasons to change from within—like we just did in chapter 4—you can draw out, notice, and reinforce your own change talk. Also, in chapter 3, we learned the skill of mindful awareness, which can help you be intentional in slowing down your thought process to take it all in. Remember, our brains fire so rapidly that sometimes it feels like thinking is automatic and outside our conscious awareness until we're able to slow down and really access it. A skillful communicator can slow that process down, noticing both sides of the ambivalence rather than focusing on just the one side that might be showing up. Maybe you've decided you need to focus on work-life balance (like Dr. X), and every time you make a move to focus more on your personal life, you hear yourself arguing for the side of staying the same: Yes, *but I need to perform at work… or I can't leave work at 5. This would never get done.* This is "stuck talk" rearing its unpretty head. You can ask yourself a question like *What would it be like for me to get home at a reasonable hour? What would change?* and then listen to the other side of ambivalence: *I could have dinner with my family* or *I would make it to my kid's softball game* or *I would get to sleep at a reasonable time.* In this chapter, we'll talk about how to deepen those responses so you are generating stronger, more powerful change talk. Ultimately, using the skills we'll review here, you can go from "I think I can" to "I do."

In this chapter we are going to talk about (1) how to help yourself; (2) how to talk with others about your change and share some ideas with them on how to best help you, including asking others to change the way they talk to you about your change; and (3) maybe even (gasp!) how to help other people change. The skills contained in this chapter are the other ingredients in the MI secret sauce, alongside MI spirit and change talk.

Who's in Your Circle?

If you've made it this far in the book for your own change, this chapter will help you with one of the biggest levers for change: engaging others around you to support your change. And if you've picked up this book to help a loved one make a change, this is a great chapter to think through how to have those conversations more effectively. Many people want to help people. You, for instance, might volunteer in your community, help at a school, or be a person others call when they're down. While many people fancy themselves as helpers, what gets missed is consideration of how important the communication around that help is. The "how" of communication is key to your success in making and sustaining behavior change—and the big bonus is that what you learn here can help you communicate more effectively with anyone about anything. That is a big promise and I will stand behind it.

To set yourself up for success on our current journey—helping you make a change that's in line with your values so you're really living the life you want to live—take a second to think about whom in your network you might want to enlist to help you change. Maybe you'll even ask some of the most important members of your support team to look at this chapter with you. How people talk to you is really important, and you can ask them to talk to you in a way that makes it more likely that you'll succeed. You might already be leaning on people as you set about implementing your simple goal from chapter 3. Fantastic! Make some quick notes here all the same.

Which people in your life have you enlisted, or do you want to enlist, in support of the changes you're currently making?

_____   _____

_____   _____

_____   _____

_____   _____

_____   _____

How do you want these folks to help you? Think back to your Change Master of the Past from chapter 2. How did other people play a factor in your successful behavior change? What help and support could you use with your current behavior change target? Take a best guess for now. Like everything, we'll use this as an opportunity to test and learn, and you can edit, revise, add to this as you work through your journey.

_____

_____

_____

_____

_____

How do you communicate your needs with these people generally? How do your conversations typically go? In what ways have you communicated successfully to enlist help in your prior change efforts? What would you like to be different?

_____

_____

_____

_____

_____

Now—how do you talk to yourself generally? What did you notice in your change talk work in the last chapter, or what have you noticed in general in your life? In what, if any, ways would you want to change how you talk to yourself, especially the motivational or self-critical parts of it?

_____

_____

_____

_____

Putting Your OARS in the Water

Let's start with some basic communication skills, represented by an acronym we MI folks often use: OARS. O stands for open-ended questions (vs. close-ended questions). A is for affirmations, R is for reflections, and S is for summaries.

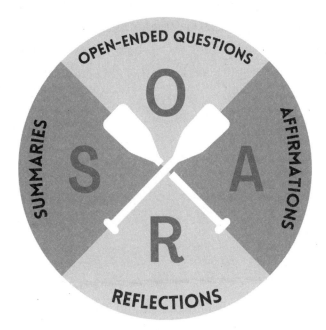

As we like to say in MI, putting your OARS in the water will help draw out and reinforce change talk and help guide you in the direction of your values and goals. So, we'll spend some time in each part of the OARS and make sure we have a good understanding of these communication skills and how best to leverage them in your change journey. These are tools that clinicians, coaches, and leaders use in effective communication—and that will help you continue to support yourself and to communicate your change more effectively with others. What's more, you've already been using some of these skills with yourself. Look back on the questions you've answered in this book; they are mostly open-ended. You've been asked to reflect. Here you'll learn the skills of how to do it for yourself—creating powerful, evocative questions; reinforcing your own change talk; and reflecting on your strengths and values with affirmations. These are the tools of the behavior science trade that create a more powerful change journey. We're going to delve into the components of OARS (just not in order completely).

Open-Ended (aka Open-Minded) Questions

Distinguishing between open- versus close-ended questions sounds simple, and you might be wondering why we make this point in MI. By definition, an open-ended question is one that cannot be answered with yes/no ("Did you exercise today?") or a data point ("How tall are you?"). Questions that are open-ended are more open-minded—they're framed in a way that allows a more open response set than close-ended questions. Open-ended questions provide more autonomy to respond in a way that is consistent with where the respondent's mind is at. Questions framed this way implicitly query the respondent's thoughts and feelings and often lead to other questions or more and different details.

Let's see how this comes to life. Your kid had a test in school today; you can ask any of the following questions when they come home:

- Did you pass the test?

- Did the test go okay?

- How did the test go?

- How was your day?

Think about the different answers you might get and how the conversation might go depending on which question you lead with. Which questions feel more open-minded to you? "Did you pass the test?" puts some pressure on the conversation; it might have implied meaning, like "You had better have passed the test, mister!" And, on the other extreme, "How was your day?" doesn't ask specifically about the test; in that case, your mind is open to whatever your kid's answer will be. When we close our questions, we narrow down the possibilities to learn and understand where someone's mind is at—we're pre-defining where the answer will go. We're also in danger of the question-answer trap, where it becomes an interview or interrogation and not a conversation. No one likes to be interrogated, and if we're going to engage others effectively in your change journey, working with them and communicating in a helpful way is going to be key. And as you know from our discussions of self-compassion and change talk, if you're going to support *yourself* in your change journey, you'll need to communicate with yourself in the same helpful way.

Let's try an exercise to really sharpen the distinction between open- and close-ended questions. Go through each question and circle whether it's an open- or close-ended question.

Did you eat sweets today?	OPEN	CLOSED
Are you okay?	OPEN	CLOSED
Do you understand?	OPEN	CLOSED
Can I help you?	OPEN	CLOSED
Have you taken your meds today?	OPEN	CLOSED

Okay. That was a bit of a trick exercise. Those are *all* close-ended questions. Let's try to open 'em up. How could you have an open mind and ask these questions more open-endedly?

Did you eat sweets today?

Open-minded version: _____

Are you okay?

Open-minded version: _____

Do you understand?

Open-minded version: _____

Can I help you?

Open-minded version: _____

Have you taken your meds today?

Open-minded version: _____

How did you do? That's an open-ended question by the way. It's not easy, or natural, to ask open questions. We're accustomed to asking close-ended questions. If you found yourself struggling, here are some helpful tips for opening up your questions. Start with "How," "What," "In what ways," or "Why"—all words that evoke experience and get you to consider not just what did or didn't happen, or what is or isn't true, but what something was like. Or say stuff like "Say more," "Tell me about...," and "Describe..." (which count as open-ended questions because they reflect curiosity in the same way).

CLOSE-ENDED QUESTION	OPEN-ENDED QUESTION
Did you eat sweets today?	How did today go? What did you eat today?
Are you okay?	How are you doing? What are you feeling?
Do you understand?	What are you taking away from this? What do you understand? What have I missed that might be helpful to you?
Can I help you?	How can I be helpful? What's the best way I can make a difference for you?
Have you taken your meds today?	How are you doing? How are things going with your meds?

Pro tip: You can use open-ended questions with yourself as a simple daily check-in. "How am I doing?" will help you dive deeper into yourself than "Am I okay?" It broadens the ask in a powerful, yet simple way.

Reflections

You'll see we're jumping right to the "R" part of OARS here—because the way you use reflections is a key skill for the "S" part (the summaries) and the "A" part (the affirmations) of OARS, which we'll cover below. A reflection is a short statement that lets someone know that you are listening and reflects back your understanding.

I often preach, "Listen, *really* listen" to patients (especially romantic partners), friends, colleagues, "And don't just sit quietly waiting to talk." Here is why it is mission critical: communication is tough! And even if we think we are amazing communicators, communication is a two-way street—that is, it's not just about what we say, but also about what the other person hears, and what they wish to express and whether we're hearing that. In this way, the ability to reflect to the people we're speaking with what we're hearing—and have them correct us if need be—helps us understand that communication is happening on both sides of the street, and how. You can even do this with yourself like you did in chapter 4, where you recorded your responses and then reflected on them. It will help you slow down and make sure you are getting to the core of what is going on for you and not just whizzing by.

Thomas Gordon (n.d.) articulated the process of communication pretty well. It's depicted in this figure.

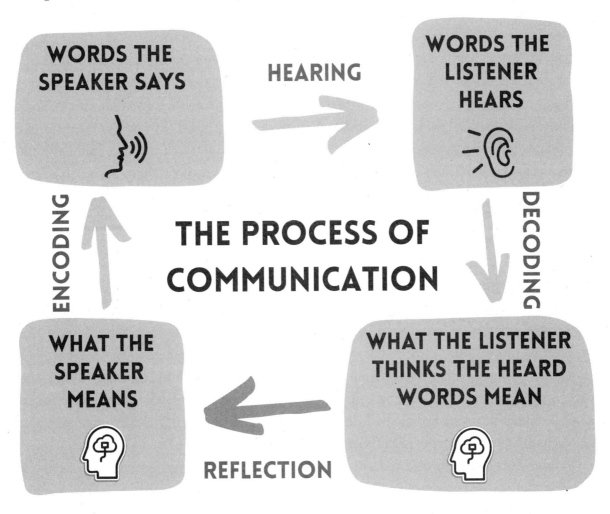

Here is my no-nonsense version of it: When I want to communicate (even like my typing right now), my mind has an idea of what I want to say/communicate. I then say it (or type it) to the intended audience/listener (you in this case), and then the listener interprets what they heard or read. Here's the bonkers thing—there are three places this can all go wrong. (These are the lighter gray arrows in the figure; each is an opportunity for miscommunication to happen.) I may have the best of intentions of communicating something amazing and really important, and what comes out of my mouth (or what my fingers type) doesn't land on it in the way I had intended, and I may not have even realized it! Or, maybe I did it perfectly well and you heard or read it wrong. Whoops! Happens to the best of us. Maybe you missed a word or you took it in a different context than I intended. A reflection helps a listener connect back to the speaker and see how the words they heard and understood relate to what the speaker actually meant or intended to communicate.

Miscommunication also happens with ourselves and our thoughts. Slowing down the process and being mindfully aware of what we're thinking on all aspects of our change journey is going to be important—this process can even help us understand ourselves better.

So, a reflection helps clarify what your mind intended to communicate and what your listener understood. Remember the old game of "telephone," where person one whispers something to another, who whispers it to another, who whispers it to another, and then eventually the person at the end says aloud what they heard, and you compare what they heard to what person one actually said? It's a barrel of laughs, and the reality is that this happens all the time in our brains. We miscommunicate and/or misunderstand. Reflections bridge that gap without asking a ton of questions. They allow you to have a flowing conversation as opposed to that question-answer trap we talked about before.

Reflections can also help you consolidate your own thinking. You can use them to slow down the process and listen to yourself (even if it's your internal monologue) and draw out what is important and meaningful to you.

Before we do some practice, I wanted to let you know about two "levels" of reflections: simple and complex. Simple reflections are, well, simple. They are straightforward reflections of what someone says (or you think they said). They're important to let someone know they have been heard, and they don't add a lot of details or deepen the conversation in a meaningful way. One catch is that you want to avoid being an annoying parrot. Simple reflections are a step beyond active listening. You don't just say back the exact words someone said. That gets frustrating. You are, instead, capturing the essence of what they said.

On the other hand, complex reflections add something. They can reflect a feeling or they can add something or reflect something implied but not explicitly stated. Complex reflections often involve making a bit of a guess at what someone is saying or thinking. It's an educated guess and it's tapping into something implied. You know when you ask someone how they are doing and they say, "Fine," and they look miserable, like something is wrong? A complex reflection would be something like "Looks like you're having a tough time" (in a supportive, empathic tone, of course). They haven't said it and you see it, so you reflect it. The real value of complex reflections comes when you can reflect and reinforce magical change talk. Remember, the more change talk you get, the more likely you are to see change. And we know that change talk begets change talk so...if you can reflect change talk, you are likely to get *more* change talk. It has been scientifically proven. This is kind of the heart and soul of what makes MI so meaningful.

One final note: reflections are always statements. That means your voice goes *down* at the end of the reflection. If your voice goes up, it becomes a question. Here's an example:

Your friend: "I'm just not sure what I want to do at this point."

You: "You're stuck." (voice inflects down at end)

vs.

You: "You're stuck?" (voice inflects up at the end)

The first one is a complex reflection because it gives a bit more than your friend offered. The second one is a question (and a closed one at that) because the voice goes up at the end.

This may seem like a fine point, and it matters. Reflections help evoke more and keep things flowing. Making a reflection more of a question, with your intonation, risks having you and your conversation partner fall into a question-answer trap, which can feel like an assessment or an interview; your conversation partner might read doubt into your intonation and be put on the defensive. Ultimately, the more you can reflect and genuinely connect for yourself and others, the more effective the communication will be.

So, think about this. What would it be like if your change supporters didn't just ask you about your change but helped you notice your feelings, your implied meaning, the stuff you mean but haven't yet said? What if you did the same for them when they were struggling? Imagine all the change that could happen? Maybe you'd both be better for it!

Summaries

The "S" in OARS stands for "summaries." This one is obvious—summaries are a series of reflections that recount or review what has been said, in a more summative way. In MI, we use them throughout a conversation, as a check-in during a dialogue to make sure you're tracking what the speaker is saying, or at the end of a conversation to wrap up and consolidate what you have heard and learned. Here's my favorite metaphor for this: Imagine the act of listening as walking through a large grassy field with someone. When you are listening, *really* listening to someone (or yourself), each time you notice something meaningful (e.g., change talk, an important insight), it's like a beautiful flower you found in the field that you pluck and put in your pocket. You don't stop the interaction; you just hold onto the flowers. At the end of the conversation or at a meaningful juncture, you take all the flowers out of your pocket, arrange them in a strategic way (e.g., softening sustain talk, emphasizing change talk, providing affirmations) and hand them all back to the speaker in a beautifully arranged bouquet—aka summary of reflections. This is like holding up the proverbial mirror and helping someone see themself as you have observed them. Summaries can connect someone to their strengths and reinforce change talk.

In general, like reflections, you want to keep summaries short and to the point. You also want to end with something evocative and collaborative, like "What did I miss?" or "How does that fit with what you were trying to say?" or "Did I get it all?" or, my absolute favorite two-word question, "What else?"

EXERCISE: Reflect, Reflect, Reflect

Reflections are a really critical part of communication with yourself and others, so we're going to have three opportunities to practice here. It's 100% up to you which one(s) you pick. Try them all or pick one that seems like it would be helpful for you. Each is an opportunity for you to notice the power of reflections for yourself and with others.

Opportunity 1

Let's have some fun (as if you weren't already)! This exercise is inspired by one of my favorite MI trainers and authors, Dr. David Rosengren (Rosengren 2017). Find a cool interview to listen to or watch; it can be with a famous person alive or dead, a local news interview, or any interview you find. Consider picking someone fun you want to learn something about. (If this doesn't sound intriguing, skip ahead. No judgment. This is your journey, your book.)

Part 1: For the first few minutes of the interview, listen and observe. What kinds of questions is the interviewer asking? What kinds of reflections are they using? Take some notes and tally up what you hear:

# of open-ended questions	# of close-ended questions

# of simple reflections	# of complex reflections

Did you notice any summaries (reflections chained together)?

Part 2: For the next few minutes, pause the interview each time the interviewee finishes speaking, right before the interviewer starts to speak again. Practice what you would say as the interviewer instead. Try out a simple reflection or a complex one. Or ask a truly curious open-ended question. Then press play and see where your head was compared to where the interviewer went.

What did you notice?

_____

_____

_____

_____

Part 3: If you're game, try out a summary of what you heard. Think about what the meaningful parts of the interview were and what you might want to reflect back—the reflection highlights pulled together in a beautiful bouquet. Try that out here:

_____

_____

_____

_____

Opportunity 2

Let's try a more traditional exercise. I'm going to make some statements, and you try to generate reflections.

Me: I am tired of being tired.

You: _____ (simple reflection)

You: _____ (complex reflection)

How was that? Hard? Easy? A simple reflection is simple, so something as straightforward as "You are tired" would work. A complex reflection digs a little deeper: "You're exhausted," or even deeper, "You are ready to make a change." That last complex reflection is a hypothesis and is taking an educated guess at what I might be feeling. It's not exactly a stab in the dark and it's a small risk. If you were wrong, no worries—I'd correct you! And of course, when you're using OARS with your own self-talk, you can correct yourself; you can make a statement to test the waters and see if it aligns with your experience.

Imagine doing this with yourself. Reflecting back what "I am tired of being tired" means to you is powerful. There's a lot embedded in that one short phrase. What is in there? Reflections can bring it out.

How about trying another one?

Me: I can't believe I am back here again. Why can't I stick with this?

You: _____ (simple reflection)

You: _____ (complex reflection)

You have a smidge more to work with here. You want your reflections to be concise and help me know you're listening. A simple one might be "You're wondering how you got back here again." Yup—it's simple. A complex one could connect to some of the emotion I might be feeling, like "You're frustrated" or "You really want the change to stick this time," or, if you want to orient me to my strengths, "You're willing to persevere and try again."

We can borrow from both the research of MI and behavior science to help guide us in ways to talk to ourselves about change. Remember in chapter 1 when we were talking about being self-compassionate? Really thinking about how we talk to ourselves and how we highlight the good can help us in the change process and is a powerful tool to communicate about change. There are no right or wrong reflections. You will realize this as you try out the approach.

Opportunity 3

How about trying this live? Grab a friend or a partner and say something like "Hey. Want to be listened to? *Really* listened to?" and then do it. Listen one-mindedly. No mobile devices in hand. No TV on in the background. Just listen and practice reflecting what your friend tells you. Notice if your voice goes up when you reflect (which turns it into a question). Just be present and listen with your heart and your ears, and notice your experience of listening and reflecting what you're hearing—as well as how your friend responds to having their experience reflected in this way. Try out an interim summary or one at the end, or both.

While it feels like you might be asking for a favor when you ask someone to do this for you, this is an incredible gift. It is rare that we listen, really listen, to one another. And you'll likely find appreciation brewing on both sides when you do this exercise. Now that you've modeled good listening and reflecting for your friend, see if they will return the favor! And, since you know how to do this more effectively by reading this chapter, you can coach them to be the kind of listener you need—empathic, compassionate, mindful—and you're on your way to have more effective members of your tribe to support your behavior change.

Then, you can teach them all that you have learned and ask them to spend some time listening to you. This can create a more effective mutual helping relationship.

Affirmations

Affirmations are reflections that affirm a strength or a value for someone, like the statement "You're willing to persevere and try again" from the last section. We use affirmations to communicate support, hopefulness, and caring and to show appreciation, particularly for someone's efforts. An affirmation can help reflect and reinforce the hard work someone is doing or the success they're having, or connect them to their sense of purpose and meaning. A strong affirmation helps someone "be seen" for the good work they're doing and the strengths they have.

Here is the thing, though—you do not want to overuse affirmations or use them disingenuously. Affirmations, in the MI sense, are not meant to cheerlead or pat you on the back. "You got this!" for instance, is not an affirmation in the MI sense, not unless you've been listening to someone talk for a while and you know they really have this under control—or have been working hard yourself and know that you have the ability to make it happen. Then you can affirmatively say "You got this!"

This is an important nuance to be mindful of—an affirmation should not be a platitude, no matter how kindly or lovingly it's intended, but something considered and earned, and issued genuinely and judiciously.

For example, if you want to…

- …communicate support, hope, or caring: "This is tough for you."

- …reinforce a value: "You care about being a reliable, available parent."

- …acknowledge strengths: "You are someone who doesn't give up."

- …reinforce actions already taken: "You began by talking to others about what worked."

Try this for yourself. Think back on your journey so far. What are you proud of? What strength or value have you leaned into? Write an affirmation for yourself. If you have multiple ones, even better. You can talk to yourself using "You…" or you can say, "I am…"

Some self-affirmations might be "I am strong and determined" or "I work hard to get stuff done" or "You're caring and kind."

Your turn: _____

_____

_____

_____

IN YOUR POCKET: Pick your favorite affirmation and capture it. This is your message to yourself about what you value and what your strengths are. Keep it close to you and reference it often. You can even use it as your own personal mantra, repeating it to yourself often. We all need some genuine affirmations for ourselves!

Before we dive into how to leverage all this great communication for your change, let me share one more pro tip, on how to give—and get—advice.

Bonus: Asking Permission

People don't love unsolicited advice. In fact, sometimes they hate it. The same extends to you, in your efforts to make a change toward the life you want and to get others in your circle to help support you in your endeavors. You likely have onboard all the knowledge you need to make the change you're considering making. My dental hygienist didn't need to teach me to floss, for instance; I had been taught that my whole life. So every time they would show me, I would roll my proverbial eyes—it didn't feel helpful in motivating me to floss. The point is, sometimes we need to help others help us, and we can use the same strategies we'd use for communication generally to give others the tools they need to know how to help us more effectively.

The real pro tip to giving advice is to ask permission. Say something like "Would it be helpful if I shared my thoughts with you?" or "Do you want some advice on that?" or "Do you want to hear how others have done it before?" Or, "I know you really want to help me; would it be okay if I share how that might be most helpful to me?" People will usually say, "Sure" or "Yes" or "Of course!" and the result is that they're more open to hearing it as opposed to being bombarded with unsolicited advice that they start defending against.

In my twenty-plus-year career I have heard of only one nurse at a Veterans hospital who asked her patient, "Would it be okay if we talked about your smoking?" The Veteran answered, "No!" and the nurse essentially left it at that, asking if it would be okay if she followed up again at some point. When that same Veteran started thinking about quitting smoking several months later, do you know whom he called? That nurse who had respected his wishes and hadn't accosted him with *her* agenda—not his. He called her asking for help. People want to be treated as autonomous beings in control of their lives and want to receive advice they have asked for or are open to receiving—not advice tossed at them. It's a small but meaningful shift. Try it—with others and with yourself!

Applying This All to Your Positive Change

Now that you know all about using OARS to communicate more effectively to facilitate and rein-force change, we'll turn to learning how to leverage this for your own positive change. There are a couple of ways. First, you can ask for what you need from folks around you. That's part of how I managed to complete Week 1 of the Couch to 5K. I asked my husband and daughter for help, for support, and for the space and grace to leave the house for the thirty to forty-five minutes I needed in the mornings.

Second, you can help the people in your support system help you in ways that are helpful. Yes, you can help them help you. I remember when I lived in Philadelphia and was considering joining a gym in my neighborhood. I told the guy I was dating about my ambivalence as we were walking past the gym. He wanted to be supportive and started cheering me on. "You can do this! It's not a far walk from your house. You got this." Do you know why I remember this conversation nearly fifteen years later? Because it wasn't helpful! It was the kind of rah-rah affirmation we talked about earlier, one that felt cliché. And, it completely invalidated my experience—the ambivalence I was feeling—by making me feel like I had to justify why I hadn't joined the gym yet. And when you get in a position of defending the status quo in this way, you're less likely to change and more likely to get more stuck. My mind came up with a bunch of "yes, but…" responses to justify why I hadn't joined the gym if it was so easy, and that just made me less likely to join. He essentially helped strengthen my resolve to *not* change. Remember I said he wanted to be supportive? Poor guy just didn't know how. And, back then, I wasn't aware that I could guide him or give him feedback, with permission. Spoiler alert—he is not the man I married. The dude I spend my days with is an engi-neer whom I have educated in how best to help me. So, when I say something like "I am thinking of restarting the Couch to 5K," he will pause and think through what to reflect back to be helpful. Even something as simple as "Oh, so you've been thinking through how to make that happen" is helpful or "You've done it before. What worked last time?" There are lots of great ways he can leverage the OARS to help me. And—he needs to know *how* to do that. It's not magically innate in most of us. So sharing some of the strategies can help.

Take a moment to revisit the questions you answered at the start of this chapter about the people in your circle. If you wrote about anyone from whom you've struggled to elicit appropriate support in the past, how does what you've learned about OARS point you toward ways you can adjust your communication with this person in the future so they can be genuinely helpful in keeping you on track with the changes you hope to make? How can you ask for the help you need?

_____

_____

_____

_____

Finally, you can use these same strategies with yourself. When I found myself thinking that I wanted (needed) to be more thoughtful about my health, I stepped back and asked myself, "What has worked before?" (open-ended question). Then I made some notes of my answers (reflections), even affirming myself along the way. ("You care a lot about this. You want to be a good role model for your daughter.") Finally, I pulled it all together and made a plan (summary). You can thoughtfully turn the OARS on yourself. And *that* is the magic!

If you feel it'll be helpful, you might try doing that now—either with the simple goal or change you've been working with, or a different change you'd like to start working toward in the future, as you continue moving toward the life you want to live and the values you want it to reflect (the stuff in the buckets from chapter 2).

The open-ended question(s) you'd like to ask yourself:

_____

_____

Your answers to that question—your reflections:

_____

_____

_____

_____

Any affirmations you want to give yourself, to reaffirm the values that have brought you to this change and the strengths you know you have, and to celebrate your successes so far with the change you're contemplating:

_____

_____

_____

_____

_____

A summary—a review of all the above, including how you want to act in the future, pulled together from the previous steps you've worked through:

_____

_____

_____

_____

_____

_____

If you find this framework helpful and want to work with it further, you can visit http://www .newharbinger.com/51543 for an OARS Worksheet.

Moving Forward

Here again is a quick recap of what we learned and did in this chapter:

- Discussed the importance of communication skills and how to use them on yourself, how to ask others to use them to help you, and how you can be a change supporter with others

- Reviewed OARS, the communication skills essential to MI

- Learned about affirmations and crafted one or more for yourself

- Learned the principle of asking permission before giving advice—and how you can help others in your support network learn to practice this principle

- Thought about how to use OARS in your behavior change journey (and maybe even to help others!)

- What else are you taking away from this chapter? What stuck with you?

_____

_____

_____

In the next and last part, we pull everything together to get started with planning. It's time to really roll up your sleeves and make a sustainable plan for the life you want to be living.

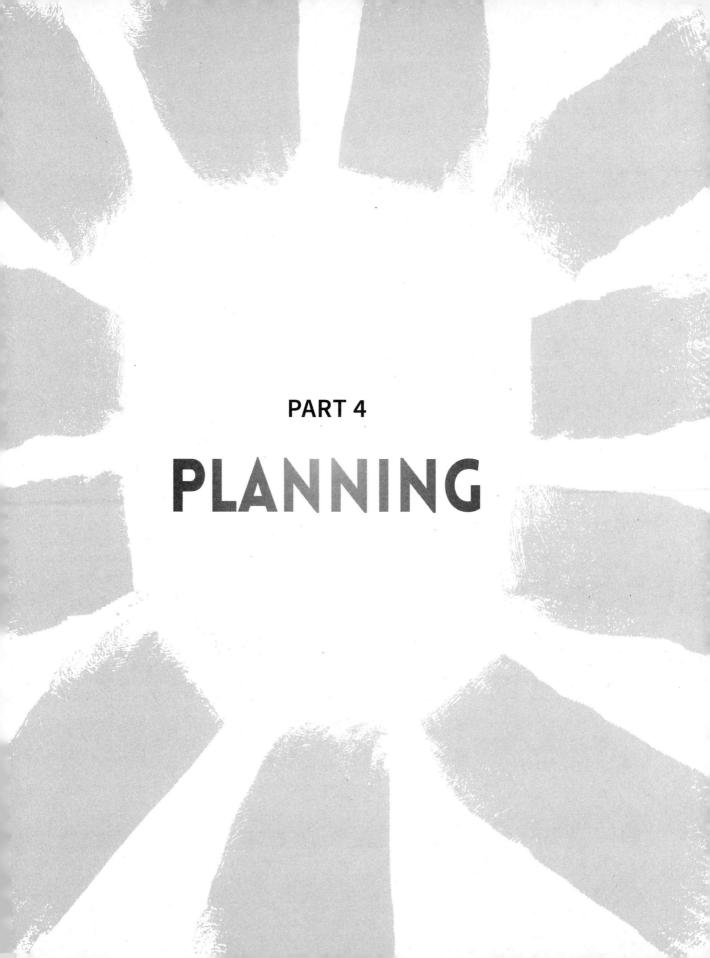

PART 4

PLANNING

CHAPTER 6

Plan

A goal doesn't just point you in a specific direction, it also pulls you in that direction.

—Ayelet Fishbach

This is the chapter you might have been waiting for all along. Sometimes it feels like positive life change should start with a plan, and yet we walked together in this book through a lot of other foundational stuff to get you pointed in the right direction and committed, *really committed*, to what you want to change. That commitment now has roots and is grounded in your values. You chose thoughtfully. You also learned about change talk and how to communicate that change most effectively to yourself and ask others to help you with OARS. If we hadn't spent that valuable time, you'd likely be running around changing a smidge here and there, never making true progress, or, sadly, you might be stuck in indecision for a long time. That is tiring and demoralizing and, well, you know how that ends—you give up. You might even have slipped back into precontemplation and forgotten that the change is anything you ever wanted. Instead, you have an identified goal and a strong "why" that will pull you as you move forward toward the life you want.

I have worked with patients who have not had their direction or plan grounded and their motivation consolidated in one direction before launching on a path. One of my favorite patients would come into sessions ready to report a new target with renewed hope for change. One time they were committed to a healthier lifestyle and had joined a food delivery service to support their change. Alas, their motivation was fleeting; they never ate the specially prepared food they ordered and lost momentum. Another time they were amped up with getting organized and invested a bunch of money in containers for organization and storage, which sat mostly empty because, well, their motivation flopped. Yet another session they showed up ready to become a fitness maven and had joined a new gym and teamed up with a friend. I was hopeful for them because I believe my patients can and will make changes, and yet something wasn't quite right. The motivation faded because they hadn't done the work we've been doing this whole book, to determine the "why" that animated the work they were doing and would keep them going even when the going got tough.

You, though, have done the necessary legwork to create sustainable change. And now, here we are, chapter 6, finally laying out your path toward change. It's time to plan! And you know why? Because you know your "why," that's why!

EXERCISE: Change Master of the Past Revisited

Before we go forward, let's go back. Revisit the Change Master of the Past exercise in chapter 2 and review what you captured when you walked through a successful change from the past. Now that you have a bit more data under your belt having done some deeper work, let's capture more info from our current vantage point.

What did you learn from the Change Master of the Past exercise? What skills and/or strengths do you already have onboard?

_____

_____

What else have you learned about yourself and your change abilities in this book so far?

_____

_____

Who are the people around you who can help you change? What can they do for you and how?

_____

_____

In what ways is your environment set up for success?

_____

_____

Based on what you have learned so far, what do you imagine you could do differently to make your change stick?

_____

_____

What might get in your way? How are you thinking you will overcome those challenges?

_____

_____

What else is on your mind? Drop some behavior science and self-knowledge here. What is coming up for you? What is in your head and your heart when you think about making this change? What have you learned that is important to you and your change journey?

_____

_____

Great job capturing all of that information. It's going to come in very handy in the rest of this chapter.

Brainstorming Pathways Toward Change

I was recently working through a planning process with a patient, whom we'll call Logan. She has been struggling with an alcohol use disorder for a long time. Being alone at night was a trigger for drinking alcohol, especially wine. And one (albeit big) glass would become a whole bottle in a night. That led to staying up late, poor sleep, and subpar performance at work. Plus, Logan's wife was not a fan of her drinking because it got in the way of things they did as a family. So, to get her on the change path toward reducing her drinking, we used a white board and drew some bubbles (just like in chapter 3); we started throwing out ideas to figure out how to reduce her alcohol use. Here's what we came up with:

- Don't buy more alcohol

- Ask wife for help and support

- Go to self-help meeting (SMART Recovery, Alcoholics Anonymous, Women in Sobriety)

- Talk to psychiatrist about changing meds and/or adding an addictions-specific medication, like naltrexone or disulfiram

- Use tools to limit alcohol consumption (e.g., set a goal and stick to it by moving objects from one pocket to another to track number of drinks)

- Talk to friends and family about what is going on

- Go to an inpatient rehab facility

- Find an accountability partner

- Give away alcohol in house

- Buy alcohol-free replacement beverages

- Find other distractions to avoid drinking late at night

- Chew gum

You see how this could go on and on. That is the point—this likely isn't your first rodeo making a behavior change, so you have lots of ideas and strategies to draw from. That is why we started this chapter by having you visit your Change Master of the Past. You have been successful in one way or another, and you can figure out how to leverage that success to fuel this one, whether the change is in the same vein or not. So now let's have you do some brainstorming.

EXERCISE: Brainstorming Session

Considering everything you captured in the above exercise, what are your possible pathways to success? How can you make this work? Your mind is likely already thinking through several options or strategies that could work for you. We're going to capture those thoughts and add a bit more. This is an initial crack at thinking through paths toward change. When we start this process, it helps to do a true brainstorm, like Logan did, where no options get rejected. Lay it out all there—bonkers options, easy options, expensive options, free options, options where you need no help, options that rely on the whole world helping you. Sky's the limit. This is brainstorming.

So capture as many ideas as come up. The goal here is quantity, innovation, and creativity. Don't write off any ideas at this stage—just notice your "yes, buts" and write the idea down anyway. What could a plan (or part of a plan) look like for you to successfully achieve the values-based behavior change you are seeking?

You can also find a more graphic brainstorming worksheet at http://www.newharbinger. com/51543. You can head over there now to check it out or use it for future brainstorming.

Evaluation Time

Now that you have several ideas, take a moment to reflect on each one and get a little judgy. What are some of the good things and not-so-good things about each potential pathway or plan? Use your critical thinking hat. Think about how hard or easy this plan would be to pull off—and think about how values-consistent it is. Is it going to get you to your goal and help you create the life you want?

Returning to Logan's case, let's see how she evaluated her possible pathways toward change. She wanted to decrease the amount of alcohol she was drinking so she could sleep better and be a better colleague and wife. One of her ideas, going to an inpatient rehab facility for a month, would probably help, as it would comprehensively address the problem. And it was too much for her at that point—it would take her away from work and family and she wasn't ready for that level of commitment, or for complete abstinence, either. Like many patients I work with, Logan's goal wasn't to stop drinking but to reduce her use in order to minimize the negative side effects—an approach we sometimes call "harm reduction" or "moderation." It's often a place individuals want to start with behavior change when they're not ready for abstinence or a "cold turkey" move. And I respect their wishes—these are their goals we're identifying and working on, not mine. (It's also true that going cold turkey from alcohol can be dangerous for a lot of folks without professional help.)

That said, Logan was open to medications that would work to reduce her craving and drinking, so we talked through what that might look like for her and some of the related pros and cons. She also had accompanied a friend who had struggled with substances to self-help groups and understood the value of a community. And yet she wasn't sure a 12-step group was the right fit for her—again, the abstinence thing was a challenge, as most 12-step groups lean heavily toward abstinence. We talked about alternatives, like SMART Recovery. We continued evaluating the options and even added a couple of ideas along the way.

Now it's your turn. Using the table below, evaluate each of the pathways for change you generated in the last exercise. Go one by one and allow yourself to imagine what that pathway would look like for you by answering the questions in each column.

PATHWAY	HOW DOES THIS FIT INTO MY VISION OF MY BEST SELF?	WHICH OF MY VALUES ALIGN WITH THIS PATHWAY?	HOW DOABLE IS THIS PATHWAY FOR ME? HOW LIKELY AM I TO DO IT?

As you were filling out the table, did your mind wander to where you ultimately want to start? Jot some initial thoughts down.

_____

_____

Choosing a Wise-Minded Starting Point

This needs to be said: there is no perfect place to start, no perfect moment to start. Motivation does not come from a magic potion, the wave of a wand, or some Genie's bottle. Organizational psychologist Dr. Adam Grant, professor at the Wharton School, said, "Many people procrastinate because they are waiting for their motivation to rise. They forget that getting started is what leads their motivation to rise" (Grant 2022). In a similar vein, one of my patients who had been struggling with several behavior changes in their life had this epiphany: "Perfect moments don't exist." And the next day they embarked on their nicotine-free journey, armed with nicotine replacement gum, a fun app to track "nicotine-free" time and how much money they were saving, and lots of support from friends and family. They realized that waiting for the perfect moment to change was a trick they were playing on themselves.

Many of us play this game on an annual basis. Ever make a New Year's resolution? What is so magical about the clock turning midnight and the calendar changing from one day to the next? Nothing. Okay, I will maybe give you that it's a "fresh start" and there's the social aspect of change—"everyone is doing it" (and the gym gets busy because so many people resolve to re-engage in their fitness journey). Most New Year's resolutions fail. Why? Because those folks haven't done the work you're doing here in this book; they haven't laid the foundation by exploring their values, thoughtfully choosing their targets, finding a pathway to change that is most likely to work, and utilizing specialized skills and knowledge to keep themselves on track. Their impulsive change is on shaky ground. New Year's resolutions *might* work and, here, we have armed you in a way to lead to more success by giving you the tools to do it over and over again because, after all, behavior change is a journey, not a one-stop destination.

For starters, I'm going to encourage you to revisit the Wise Mind skill we reviewed in chapter 2. Remember Reasonable Mind (data, facts, information) and Emotion Mind (feelings, mood) and how they come together to find Wise Mind? When you narrow in on your starting point, use your Wise Mind to help you select one that both makes rational, logical sense and feels right. We're going to pick an initial starting point that feels wise minded to you and put it to the test.

Go back to your evaluations and think through what is doable. One way to think about this is by answering the question "What has worked for you before?" (You can answer with either an exact plan or the gist of it.) For me, when I start my healthy lifestyle journey (repeatedly), I often start with tracking my food. It's a good foundational place for me to raise my awareness of what I am eating (quantity and quality). It helps remind me that almonds are a protein-rich power food I can turn to, and that I only need a few of them. This tracking strategy—a version of what's called self-monitoring in the behavior science world—has worked well for me many times. In general, self-monitoring is one of the most effective tools you can use, and you have already done a version of it in chapter 3.

Deep breath. Maybe even close your eyes… Then open them and consider all you have written in this chapter. And then…drum roll…what is your wise-minded starting point (or initial goal)? What makes the most sense to you and feels right at the same time?

Wise-minded starting point: _____

_____

_____

Next, envision yourself doing what you listed above for your wise-minded starting point. What do you need to make this plan happen? What tools and resources do you need to accomplish it?

_____

_____

_____

_____

_____

How ready do you feel with this particular plan? _____

| 0 | 1 | 2 | 3 | 4 | 5 | 6 | 7 | 8 | 9 | 10 |

NOT AT ALL   NEUTRAL   COMPLETELY
READY   READY

Why did you pick that number and not 0?

_____

_____

Finally, how much does this plan feel like a good place to start for you? _____

```
┌─────────────────────────────────────────────────────────────┐
│  |   |   |   |   |   |   |   |   |   |   |                    │
│  0   1   2   3   4   5   6   7   8   9   10                   │
└─────────────────────────────────────────────────────────────┘
```

NOT AT ALL   **NEUTRAL**   **COMPLETELY**

Why did you pick that number and not 0?

_____

_____

IN YOUR POCKET: This is a good moment to stop and capture your wise-minded starting point or goal. You might take a picture of what you just wrote above, or use the space below to create something—words, a drawing, whatever—that will serve as a reminder of your goal so you don't forget it and you get inspired by it. This is an important moment in your change journey.

Climbing the Change Mountain

Now that you have your wise-minded starting point in hand, take a step back and let's envision the change journey. It's not likely to be a straight path. We'll talk more in the next chapter about how to stay engaged and motivated as you move through it; for now, we'll start with accepting what the journey will look like.

Have you ever hiked up a mountain? Or, can you imagine what hiking up a mountain is like? You start at the bottom and you work your way up. Most mountain hiking trails involve switch-backs. You climb up and over and then you "switch back" and climb up and over the other way, always on a slight incline, always moving upward. Think of a zigzag pattern. Sometimes, in the middle of the climb, it feels arduous and tiring, like you aren't progressing at all—like you haven't moved an inch upward and will be hiking for forever. Yet, from across the valley, if I were watching you, I would see the progress you are making moving up and toward the summit. When you are in the throes of a change process, it is not linear and might not always feel easy. It could feel like you're not moving forward and making progress when, really, you have made significant gains; you're just not yet in a position to see them. Keeping this perspective in mind can help when you're getting tired and your mind starts to tell you it's not working. Pull back and check your progress.

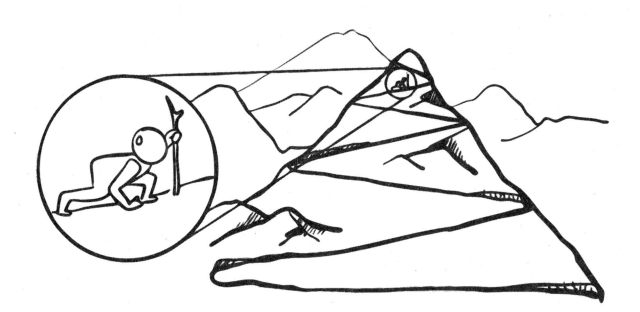

Remember the Simple Goal Tracker from chapter 3, the tool you have to check your progress? You can use a version of it to track your new wise-minded goal. This self-monitoring will help keep you honest with yourself by noticing what isn't working and what is. Both are important. Giving yourself credit for your gains is just as important as noticing where you're struggling and where you might need to shift your plan to be more successful.

We started with a simple tracker. At this point, if you find it helpful and it feels like a good fit for you, you can add some other info to that tracker. Logan, for instance, would often misuse alcohol when she was stressed or not feeling great. Adding a simple mood tracker helped us identify a pattern and when she might be at a higher risk for drinking or overdrinking (more than her goal). I included a version below, which you can also find at http://www.newharbinger.com/51543, to give you an idea of what this could look like for you. You also can track your wise-minded goal and other stuff using a planner or a calendar (electronic or old-school paper). If you have a system that already works for you, use it and add to it.

WISE-MINDED GOAL AND MOOD TRACKER

WISE-MINDED GOAL:

	DAY	MOOD	GOAL PROGRESS
○	MON		
○	TUES		
○	WED		
○	THURS		
○	FRI		
○	SAT		
○	SUN		

WHAT WORKED:

WHAT STILL NEEDS WORK:

It also might be helpful to plot out what your change mountain might look like. You can put your vision of your Best Self—the vision of life that all your wise-minded starting points are leading you to—at the top. And then consider: which smaller valued goals do you see yourself wanting or needing to achieve along the way to that summit?

Use the space below to draw your mountain. Include the trail leading up to the summit if you like—some of the switchbacks you might need to navigate as you make your way to the top. Also include some of the values and affirmations you see yourself using to motivate yourself along the way. You might even draw these things as little signposts you see along your mountain trail, getting you through those switchbacks and the obstacles you'll inevitably encounter. You can even get extra creative and depict the whole mountain range, with all the changes in your journey, each as a separate mountain, so you can zoom out and see the life you are working on creating, kinda like you saw in the drawing above.

Moving Forward

Here's a recap of what we learned and did in this chapter:

- Revisited our Change Master of the Past in preparation for planning

- Did some serious brainstorming and then evaluated all the many paths you could take to get to your goal

- Selected a wise-minded goal

- Reviewed the value of self-monitoring (aka tracking) and discussed adding some addition information, like mood

- Explored climbing a mountain as a metaphor for our change journey and then sketched some of that journey, thinking through your tools and skills to help you succeed

- What else? What are you taking away from this chapter? Take some notes about what stuck with you.

_____

_____

_____

Now that you have your vision of your mountain in front of you—and the Best Self, the life you want, that awaits you—take a moment to appreciate all the skills you have to help you make this journey. Mindfulness, self-compassion, a sense of your most important values, the ability to plan goals and track progress toward those goals, the power to understand your own change talk and how to motivate yourself, the ability to enlist others to help motivate you when you need it... there are so many!

Of course, there are a few more skills we can learn to help you get and stay on track. In the next chapter, we'll look at tools that will help you sustain behavior change once it's begun and get yourself back on track when old patterns rear their heads—as they will! This final chapter is an important one. Let's dive in.

CHAPTER 7

Staying Engaged and Maintaining Your Motivation

The [hu]man on top of the mountain didn't fall there.

—Vince Lombardi

So here you are. At the end of this book. Where are you in your journey toward change? You picked up this book and made it this far for your own reasons. What were they? Take a moment to visit with your original "why." What brought you here? Staying connected to your reasons, the original ones or the ones you discovered along the way, can help keep that motivation going.

You've added so much to that original "why" throughout this journey. Now think through your reasons for change again. What is your current "why"? Your "why" may change as you experience the new you—the change itself can help uncover new reasons for change that you didn't recognize or even know would be possible.

And here you are, still reading these words. There is lots of evidence that you care. You want to make a change and, sometimes, wanting isn't enough to make the change happen. There can be a gap between what we intend to or want to do and what winds up happening. Ugh! It's so frustrating sometimes, how stuff gets in the way. You might have even walked away from an exercise or chapter in this book so sure you were going to make it happen and then—bam!—something caught your attention and drove you off course. Maybe it was even something unavoidable.

I felt this way at the beginning of the COVID-19 pandemic. I had gotten into a fantastic gym routine. I was running (well, my version of running) regularly and felt strong and in charge of my life—in control. You should have seen me and my big smile at the gym. As soon as the pandemic hit and social distancing was in place, everything changed—all of a sudden I wasn't allowed to be near non-family humans, let alone go to the gym. I was so bummed. I had to have a serious talk with myself and remind myself of what was important to me (my "why")—being healthy and feeling strong and in charge—and then I brainstormed ways to continue to make the change happen in that new socially distanced world, just like we did in the last chapter. I jumped on some fitness bandwagons to try them out and did yoga from my bedroom with my then puppy crawling all over me. I started walking and running outside, where it was "safe." I kept the behavior change going. I knew, in that moment, my motivation was shaky and it was "make it or break it" time. I made it, at least that time.

The COVID-19 pandemic was a worldwide crisis that people had to work around. It was life-changing for the entire world—it was a big deal. There are often much smaller, less threatening deals that get in our way. Maybe you're a parent or caretaker who has a boatload of competing priorities. Maybe you have a demanding job with a demanding boss. Maybe you struggle with depression or anxiety. Behavior change is hard, and sustaining behavior change is often even harder than starting it. That is what we are going to spend time on in this chapter: figuring out how to keep engaged in your change journey and re-engage when you need to, by understanding how to utilize rewards, navigate triggers that might come up on your way, tap back into your own motivation and capacities for change when you need to, and more.

Rewards

What are your thoughts about why staying the course is harder than starting it? How do you usually feel when you get started on a behavior change journey? Maybe you are like I was, all smiley at the gym, feeling proud, enjoying the energy from the changes I was making. People were complimenting me and I was feeling good. In behavior science terms, these are all referred to as reinforcers, things that bolster and help you continue your behavior, like a sticker chart where you get a sticker each time you accomplish something, or like a treat I gave my puppy each time she did the behavior I was looking for.

Rewards are a powerful component of the behavior change process. So let's plan for you to notice or create some rewards. While behavior change can be hard, we usually gain some of the intended benefits from that change—feeling more energized and clearheaded from getting to sleep on time; breathing better from smoking less; climbing a flight of stairs without getting winded because you're exercising more. Let's look at this together to see how we can get your awareness muscle noticing the rewards that come your way and perhaps create rewards and incentives to fortify your process.

Visit your Change Master of the Past (chapter 2) and remember how it felt to make the change. What did you gain from it? What felt good? What else changed besides your behavior? What were the proverbial stickers on your sticker chart? What kept you motivated and engaged? What was rewarding about that behavior change? Write some of these rewards down:

_____

_____

_____

_____

Now shift to thinking about your current behavior journey. What would be or is rewarding from your behavior change? Think about this a different way—what are some of the good things about the change you are making? How does it (or would it) make you feel? How has it changed (or could it change) your life for the better? What surprises did you find in changing your behavior? If you need inspiration, refer back to the Miracle/Magic Question in chapter 4. Jot some notes down about some of the positive changes you're noticing, or what might happen once you make the change you're planning to make, if you haven't gotten there yet.

_____

_____

_____

_____

If you're struggling to think through what is rewarding about your behavior change, that's a good indicator that you could be in danger of losing the oomph to keep going with the change journey. In that case, you might have to intentionally create reinforcers for yourself. A great example of this is starting an exercise routine. It can be tough to get started and to keep going—finding the time, the energy, the opportunity can be hard. One strategy people sometimes use is to allow themselves to only watch their favorite show while they are working out. So they stream the show only while on the treadmill or elliptical, for example, or listen to their favorite podcast only while out walking. Or, for people who thrive on social relationships, they enlist others to help them with the behavior or buddy up to do the behavior together because part of the reward becomes the social interaction.

These are just a few examples of creating a reward or incentive for yourself. There are tons more. You can use social media surfing as a reward—give yourself thirty minutes to scroll through Facebook or Instagram only after you have spent thirty minutes on the work you have been avoiding (reducing procrastination is another change folks often work on). You can take yourself shopping for a special treat to reward yourself for the hard change you're doing. Of course, rewards are personal; what might be rewarding to me might not be a good fit for you. This is an important moment to think through how to personalize your journey, which is never "one size fits all."

You can also gamify your rewards by setting them according to a structure and making it fun. For example, you might challenge yourself to do the behavior three days in a row for a bonus reward. You can try breaking down the journey into steps and give yourself points or rewards for each part of it you complete. Think about your favorite game and how you can use some of those principles. Imagine you are trying to be more outgoing and interact more at parties, meetings, and other social events. You might give yourself points for each interaction you attempt—maybe even more points for more meaningful interactions—like 10 points for a party and 1 point for saying "thank you" to your mail carrier. And then pick a point target (e.g., 100 points) for buying yourself a treat to celebrate your progress.

What are some additional rewards you could add? One of my roommates used to treat herself with a piece of high-quality chocolate whenever she finished a page of her dissertation. Writing her dissertation was onerous for her and yet being a professor was important, so she wanted to stick with it. Treating herself with some yummy chocolate did the trick to get her through, one page at a time.

How can you treat yourself for the hard work of behavior change? What are some ways to give yourself the proverbial (or literal) sticker on the sticker chart? What do you find rewarding that you can add to your journey to incentivize yourself?

_____

_____

_____

_____

Reality check time. When we make a change, we might also lose something to make space for that change. We usually have to give up or shift something that we might notice missing. When I am fully committed to a healthier lifestyle, I miss regularly having sweets and baked goods—donuts are always a tough one for me. Not being able to have sweets whenever I want them feels like a loss, even though it isn't consistent with my values and goals of being healthy. Similarly, when someone makes the decision to reduce or stop drinking alcohol, they miss it. They notice the absence—sometimes even just of holding a particular glass in their hand or of the feeling alcohol provides—and need a strategy for replacement. And for someone who's working toward their dream of being an artist or a writer, well, that decision might also involve some loss—say, the loss of stability that might be associated with the job they're giving up; the loss of social time spent with friends and family as they devote more of their energy to achieving their own goals. And your hard work usually isn't rewarded right away.

This is a moment to think through what some of the not-so-good things about your behavior change are. What will you miss? What do you miss already? This is an important question and one we need to be thoughtful and honest about because if we don't address and plan for it, that "missing" sometimes can get in the way of sustained behavior change and the life you want to be living.

In a similar vein, sometimes our behavior change plan itself feels tough to do and has its own not-so-good aspects. Maybe you feel like you don't have the time or you aren't a morning person and can't get up earlier to make the change happen if that was part of your plan (like flossing or working out in the morning). Similarly, maybe you really want to work on your sleep and you enjoy the quiet at night after everyone in the house has gone to bed; so while you want to improve your sleeping, you will miss staying up late. Or, maybe you really want to cut down on social media scrolling and worry about missing out on what is going on in the world (FOMO—fear of missing out—can be strong). And, the big one: maybe the plan to make a change also makes you anxious, and you haven't yet changed this behavior because avoidance (not changing) is comfortable. This happens a lot with people who have social anxiety or depression. On one hand, they feel safe staying away from social gatherings, in the comfort of their own home. On the other hand, they are missing out on important parts of their lives, things they really value, like feeling connected to loved ones. Sometimes we have to help ourselves navigate the short-term costs tempered with the long-term gains. Behavior change is complicated, and understanding what forces are at work can help us fortify your plan.

What do you suspect might get in the way or what might you miss with your behavior change plan?

_____

_____

_____

Now let's step back and look at the pros and cons of changing and not changing (aka staying the same) in one simple 2x2 grid. Folks find an exercise like this helpful to remind them of the full picture when they find their mind stuck on one quadrant or another. It can stimulate mindful awareness of your full journey and help ground you in what is important.

PROS OF NOT CHANGING	CONS OF NOT CHANGING
CONS OF CHANGING	**PROS OF CHANGING**

We're going to start in the top left box (Pros of Not Changing) and fill in each box, going in the reverse-clockwise direction.

Pros of Not Changing: Be honest here and look at what you have written above and have been thinking about throughout our time together in this book. What are some of the good things about staying the same? What has kept you stuck? You are a rational human and have been stuck not changing—that's probably why you picked up this book—so what are some of the reasons you haven't yet changed? Put that in this box.

Cons of Changing: This is where you're going to capture some of your hesitation for making the change, giving up the behavior, and enacting the change plan. What do you perceive as some of the challenges related to changing?

Pros of Changing: What can you imagine will be different when you make your change? Think back to chapter 4 and the Miracle/Magic Question. What will be the positive differences in your life when you fully make the change?

Cons of Not Changing: Now, what made you pick up this book in the first place? What was getting in the way of the life you want to be living? What are some of the cons of staying the same? If you decided to not change and to stay stuck, what would that look like for you and your life?

Here is what this might look like for someone who would like to procrastinate less and get their work done in a timelier manner instead of waiting to the last minute, losing sleep to meet deadlines, and so on:

PROS OF NOT CHANGING	CONS OF NOT CHANGING
• More "free" time • Watch *The Office*	• Make mistakes • Lose sleep • Panic • Always worrying • Miss out on stuff and still not getting work done
CONS OF CHANGING	**PROS OF CHANGING**
• Have to plan more • Miss out on fun events	• Less anxiety • Better results (grades) • Time to review/revise • Fewer errors

Pull back and look at your 2x2 grid. During your change journey, your mind will wander to the left column, and you will hear yourself say or think things like "My life isn't so bad" or "I like things about my life," or you might find yourself feeling like "Change is impossible" or "Making this change is scary." All those thoughts and feelings are important, valid ones. This is where some of the tools you're putting in your toolbox—self-compassion and values (chapter 1) and mindfulness (chapter 3)—are going to be essential.

You're also going to use those tools to turn intentionally to everything in the right column. The life you want to be living is different and could be better, and your current path is causing you some level of suffering or challenge. You want to make this change and create a life that is more consistent with your values. Holding what you wrote in the right column is going to keep you connected to all of that.

Everything in this 2x2 grid is true for you; accepting and validating that is important, and allowing your mind to stay stuck on the left side is going to keep you stuck *not* changing. Be aware of that and intentionally move your thoughts to the right side of the grid—the right side of change.

IN YOUR POCKET: This is another opportunity to grab a part of this book and keep it with you "in your pocket." Which parts of the 2x2 grid would be most helpful for you to carry around and review? Some people find it validating to see the whole thing—all four boxes—laid out, while some like to focus on the right column only. Maybe you'd like to rewrite the 2x2 grid in colors or embolden some words. When I used to do this with groups, we would write some words in big letters to indicate just how important those reasons were, and write other words smaller to indicate they were less important. So, take a pic of what you created above or re-create it in a manner that feels helpful to you and consider keeping it "in your pocket."

Triggers

"I am so triggered" or "That is such a trigger for me." Ever hear someone say something like that? Ever hear yourself say that? A trigger is something that elicits an unwanted behavior or emotional reaction. In the world of substance use, a trigger might be something that elicits a craving, making someone think about using a substance. This is what is meant when people talk about "people, places, and things,"—those can be triggers, posing a high risk for the recurrence of the behavior a person is trying to change. It's not limited to the temptations for alcohol or drugs, of course. When you walk past a restaurant and the scent of the most delicious food wafts into your awareness and overwhelms your senses, what happens? You might have not been hungry before, but now, suddenly, the scent works as a trigger: you are thinking about eating, your mouth might be watering, and maybe you find yourself stopping and heading in to sample the deliciousness, without even being 100% aware of the process that happened. It's not unconscious; you are awake and aware. And yet a lot of this can happen so quickly that intervening is challenging—not impossible, just hard.

On your change journey, triggers will likely come up for you—experiences that steer you back to "old" behaviors or to choices that lead you off your chosen path. One way to get ahead of this is to think through some of those triggers now, what might get in the way of your successful behavior journey. Awareness is power. If you know what can put you at risk, you can cope or plan for it.

EXERCISE: Your Triggers

Triggers can be anything. We're going to capture some of the more obvious ones for you, which will set you up to be on the lookout for additional triggers as you continue your change journey. We'll start with some broad categories of triggers. I encourage you to think about the past and present and consider internal (within your own mind and body), external (in your environment), and interpersonal (with other people) triggers. Think about triggers as "high risk" situations for you—they put you at risk of not meeting your goals or acting in line with your values.

Some internal triggers we will look at are thoughts and feelings. When I'm tired or stressed or even bored, I'm often triggered to go off my healthy journey. I might even hear myself saying, *You deserve that* _____ (candy, cake, something inconsistent with my goals). I try hard not to keep those kinds of foods in the house because when they're around, I find myself reaching for them without even thinking about it. Keeping candy around is a trigger for me—a "thing" that puts me at risk for not acting in line with my values and goals.

Similarly, people and social situations can be triggers to consider. Who might be a trigger for you and get in the way of your behavior change journey? Or what types of social situations might be higher risk for you? My patients who are working to reduce alcohol use usually have certain friends who are their drinking buddies or particular social situations (like parties or events) where drinking alcohol, using drugs, overeating, smoking cigarettes, gossiping (all things most of us want to keep in check) are more likely. When I was working on eating healthier, my Italian grandmother used to be a trigger because she lived up to the stereotype by showing you her love with food, and if you didn't eat "enough" (which was a *lot*) she would push more food on you. I had to learn to be assertive in a way that didn't offend her. So, you see, identifying someone, or being around that someone, as a trigger doesn't make those people "bad" (my sweet Nonny was amazing!); it just helps you be more aware and prepared.

Let's generate some ideas for each trigger category below.

People

Are there people who, when you're around them, might put you at risk for engaging in the behavior you're trying to change? For example, a group of friends you only hang out with when you smoke marijuana together or someone who is not supportive of your change journey in general (maybe because they are stuck doing the old behaviors)?

_____

_____

Places

Are there places that might be triggers for you? This could be a specific spot in your home or as broad as a part of the country. What are some places or settings that might be risky for you, such as those where you often engaged in the old behavior? For example, driving in the car with the window down might be a trigger for someone who used to smoke in the car, or going to a mall might be a high-risk spot for someone trying to curb their spending.

_____

_____

Things

Are there objects or things that trigger you to engage in the behavior you are trying to change? Think about what might be associated with your old behaviors. This could be as obvious as a vape cartridge if you're trying to quit vaping or a box of cookies if you're trying to eat less sugar; or as subtle as having cash in your wallet if you're trying to spend less money or if you paid for your old behaviors using cash.

_____

_____

Emotions/Feelings

Are there specific emotions that trigger you? Boredom or frustration can be triggers. Similarly, feeling rejected or betrayed might be a big trigger. Happiness and joy might also trigger engagement in the behavior you're trying to change. Also consider pain here. If you are someone who has chronic pain, would you consider being in pain a trigger that might get in the way of your change journey?

_____

_____

Thoughts

Sometimes our minds can be unkind. We have discussed our inner critic and how thoughts can show up that trigger us to feel a certain way, which can, in turn, trigger us to engage in the behavior we're trying to change. *You're a failure* or *You suck* are inner critic thoughts that can leave us feeling demoralized. When you're having these types of unhelpful thoughts, it can leave you feeling negative, which puts you at risk for the old behaviors to show back up; it's harder to be vigilant and motivated when thoughts are keeping you down.

Lots of other thoughts can be triggering. A simple thought like *Pumpkin pie is amazing and I should have some* might lead me quickly down the road of having several slices of pie even when I'm trying to make healthier choices. *F*ck it* is also a thought that can be triggering and lead you off the path of your positive change.

What are things you think or say to yourself that can be triggering? What are some things you hear your inner critic saying that can lead you off the path of behavior change you are working so hard on?

_____

_____

Activities/Events

One patient had a hard time not having a cold beer when he would mow the lawn. Mowing the lawn was so deeply associated with drinking beer that he needed a clear plan to avoid it. For others, activities as mundane as grocery shopping can lead to temptations. Maybe an activity like scrolling through social media is a trigger for you? It might expose you to cues you've been avoiding (like food or alcohol) or make you feel certain ways (FOMO). There also might be events that trigger you—celebrations like a wedding or job promotion or sad events like funerals.

What activities/events might be associated with the behavior you're trying to change and might trigger you to engage in old behaviors?

_____

_____

Others

What else might be a trigger for you? What did we miss?

_____

_____

_____

If you're having a hard time coming up with triggers, spend some mindful time noticing when you think about engaging in the behavior you're trying to change. One patient reminded themself to observe what was in their head, heart, and body by posting sticky notes saying things like "Be here now" or "Slow down" in their house and car. Another set reminders on their phone to "stop and notice." This helped raise their awareness and identify triggers for them. You can also use one of the trackers in this book to take notes often and track your triggers, looking for patterns. Consider coming back and adding to this list after trying some of these things.

Look through what you generated above; let's prioritize those triggers a bit. What triggers are you most worried about? Which ones feel like they could have power over you, that they are likely to get in the way? Note those triggers here:

_____

_____

_____

Now, you likely have some ideas or strategies in mind to manage each of these big triggers. Sometimes avoidance is the easy and obvious go-to. Staying away from certain "people, places, and things" is a great place to start. Unfortunately, that's often impossible. We can't avoid everything by living in a bubble. Social triggers are particularly hard because we can't avoid humans altogether, and that usually isn't consistent with other values. So having a plan for what to do when you're confronted with a trigger is helpful. What will you do? Mindfulness might help here. If you come face-to-face with a trigger, find your feet. Get yourself into the moment. And then stay in the moment until you feel you can mindfully navigate through the situation. Being triggered is a lot like being in Emotion Mind, disconnected from Reasonable Mind. Being aware of which state of mind you're in can help you find your wise-minded path forward. What else can you come up with to manage when you are triggered? Think about what you've learned in this book and what you've had success with:

_____

_____

_____

How was that? If you struggled at all to come up with ideas, below are some more ways to manage triggers and high-risk situations that might work for you or maybe inspire you. Read through this list and store it away for a future moment. Hey, even add to it by engaging with your in-person or online support network to ask what has worked for other people. Sometimes we learn by watching others. This is what a lot of mutual support groups are about!

These are in no particular order and, like all guidance in this book, are here for you to take what works for you and leave the rest.

- Cope ahead: If you identify a trigger or high-risk situation on the horizon, don't ignore it. Face it by coping ahead of time. Plan or strategize—ahead of time—for how you'll manage it when it shows up. For example, if you're working on trying to get to bed on time and know that a risky scenario for you is getting sucked into social media at night and mindlessly scrolling, cope ahead by putting your device to bed, too. Plug in your device across the room from the bed (or even in another room), and intentionally say goodnight to it. Or, if you know a holiday is coming up and any number of triggers will show up, depending on what you are trying to change, plan in advance. "Cope ahead" is about not being blindsided. It is accepting that a situation can be triggering and coping in advance to manage those triggers.

- Set a timer: Triggers sometimes show up unannounced; that happens more often than we would like. When they do, notice that you've been triggered and notice the urge to engage in the behavior you're trying to change. Set a timer (ten to fifteen minutes works well for this). Give yourself at least those ten to fifteen minutes between the trigger and choosing whether you'll engage in the behavior. Cravings or urges—for food, alcohol, other substances, behaviors—reliably peak and then fizzle out if you wait them out, so this is a helpful, well-grounded strategy. I do this when I have a craving for a sweet treat. If I still want it after the timer goes off, I go for it, mindfully and thoughtfully. I didn't "give in" mindlessly in those cases. It was a wise-minded choice.

- Surf the urge: Similar to setting a timer, use your mindfulness muscle to imagine the urge as a big ocean wave. Then, surf that wave, in your mind, with your body; just ride the sensations, letting them be there, without reacting to or judging them. This is an opportunity to remind yourself that you have control—not of the urge or of the trigger, but of what you choose to do, and also to create the space between the urge and engaging in the behavior.

- Create a speed bump or barrier: Once you identify a trigger, see if you can notice the well-worn path between the trigger and the behavior you're trying to change. Someone who is trying to drink less alcohol, for instance, might find themself drinking at home, alone, where they have easy access to a liquor cabinet. Maybe they don't want to totally get rid of all liquor in the house as a means of limiting their alcohol consumption, so instead, they make it harder to access it by moving it to the attic or basement or putting a lock on it. The same is true for folks who find their mobile device gets in the way of their goals; they create a speed bump by moving apps off their phones, adding app use timers, or plugging in their device across the room at night so they aren't tempted to look at it before bed or as soon as they wake up in the morning. These are examples of barriers that make the triggers harder to access and speed bumps that allow more time and space to contemplate what you really want to do and whether it is "worth it."

- Play the "tape" through: When you're confronted with a trigger and have the urge to do the thing you've been avoiding, play it out in your head. I used to be a big procrastinator, and sometimes I still have the urge to put off doing work, including writing this book. Today I blocked a chunk of time to get writing done and noticed the urge to just chill and relax and hang with the pups. I even heard myself saying stuff like *You deserve some downtime, Drapkin*. And I thought through what would happen if I blew off a whole day of writing. I might relax for a little, catch up on some shows, and then—bam!—anxiety, guilt, shame, and panic would show up when I would realize what I had done—that I'd avoided the work I had planned on and needed to get done today. Playing that through helped me see the consequences of my choices. Ultimately, I chose to chill for a couple of hours first (and I set a timer to keep myself honest) because I really did deserve some downtime before I got my fingers typing these words. I didn't let my procrastination urges win the war. Nor did I suppress them, in ways that might've made them harder to fight later. I also practiced self-compassion and didn't beat myself up. I took a moment to think about my situation and make the decision that would be best for me, the things I want to do, and even the life I want to live.

- Find an alternative and incompatible behavior: When you're at risk for doing the behavior you're trying to change, pick a behavior that is incompatible. For example, if you're trying to stop smoking or vaping, try drinking water or chewing gum. Consider behaviors that won't likely become new habits you eventually will need to change. For example, drinking coffee instead of smoking is a risky one since you will become dependent on caffeine. Have a battery of behaviors thought through to help you, in advance, so when the urge to engage in an old behavior shows up, you have a plan for what to do instead.

This is just a snippet of strategies to help you manage your thoughts, feelings, and behaviors related to triggers so those no longer control your behavior. This is also an ongoing process of learning and doing, so tracking will help you learn more about what works and doesn't work.

Which of these strategies would you be willing to try?

_____

_____

_____

What about the strategies that you chose seems like it will be most effective for you?

_____

What else have you tried that has worked when you've been confronted with triggers?

_____

_____

Which of your strengths have you used or could you use to avoid your triggers?

_____

_____

IN YOUR POCKET: What is your trigger intervention plan? What will you do to avoid triggers or manage when you are triggered? Write a few notes to your future triggered self or take a pic of something to remind you of your strategy.

Of course, no matter how good you become at anticipating triggers, controlling for them, and learning how to respond to them, it's inevitable that you'll succumb to one in time or find yourself lapsing back into old behaviors in some other way, straying from your desired path. The good news is this is totally normal; most of the evidence-based psychotherapies (e.g., cognitive behavioral therapy) we mentioned in the introduction acknowledge this as such, and what we know from these approaches helps us plan for this digression from our planned path.

HALT and Connecting with the Basics

If you're finding that some of your old behaviors have recurred, it might also be time to do a basic self-check. Are you taking care of yourself, doing the basics? The acronym HALT (hungry, angry, lonely, tired) helps you see if you're taking care of your basic needs for food, sleep, rest, and social contact. So the next time you find yourself wavering on your path to change—say in the moment you're confronted by a trigger, or after a prolonged series of actions that don't feel in line with the actions you want to be taking—literally stop (HALT) and check on how you're taking care of your basic needs:

- **Hungry:** How are you nourishing yourself? And are you mindfully eating? If you're hungry, it can impact your mood, your sleep, and your overall wellbeing.

- **Angry:** How are you doing emotionally? What challenging emotions are you experiencing? Being angry every now and then is typical. Being chronically angry or in a negative emotional state is a tough place to be. If you can't shake a negative mood, consider whether seeking professional help might be needed.

- **Lonely:** We are social organisms. How much time are you spending alone? Are you missing social connectedness?

- **Tired:** And sleep—one of the most underrated variables for our health and wellbeing. How are you sleeping? Are you getting enough sleep? Is something getting in the way of your sleep: anxiety, nightmares, or something else?

HALT is a quick way to stop and check in on those four domains. Another important variable is our old friend self-compassion. When you're feeling like it's hard to stick with the change you hope to make, consider: how kind and gentle are you being to yourself? Often when we are struggling, our inner critic shows up and starts yelling nasty things at us—*You suck* or *You are never going to get a handle on this!* Combat that critic with kindness. Give yourself a Self-Compassion Break, over and over. You're on the journey, even if it isn't going perfectly. We knew that struggles and relapses were likely; behavior change is hard business. Celebrate all your successes, no matter if you think they're small. That includes still being here, reading these words.

Managing Recurrences

When a behavior rears its ugly head and recurs, a lot of people call that "relapse." And some treatment approaches treat you as if you are back at the starting line, back at zero. Not here. We respect that recurrence is part of the process and see it as an opportunity to learn—it is not failure.

Think about how humans learn to walk. We use what we can to get around; we crawl, scoot, wiggle, and then we try to ambulate on two feet and—crash! Over and over. Each fall teaches us something: how to hold ourselves, what works and what doesn't to maintain balance. Eventually, we walk. In fact, we don't just walk; we run. *And* we still fall occasionally—because someone left something in our path, our shoelace got untied, or in a certain moment, we were clumsy. Life is the same way; there are obstacles or challenges we learn from, each of which is an opportunity to reset and move forward—not "failures," as sometimes our mind or inner critic likes to call them.

This part of the book is here to help you if you find your old behavior has slipped back into your life, or your change plan had a setback. In her memoir, Dr. Marsha Linehan, the founder of dialectical behavior therapy (DBT), provides some wisdom here: "Never give up. It doesn't matter how many times you fall; what's important is that you always get up and try again" (Linehan 2021, 124). Know and remember that you can come here when you need support getting back on your journey after a detour. Detours can look like anything—a small pitstop off your journey for a moment engaging in your old behavior or a full return to the status quo (where you started or even further backward).

When we "feel" motivated and don't follow through, negative self-talk sometimes shows up and gets in our way of doing the thing we want to do. If you're feeling dismayed, let's try to get you back on the behavior change journey page.

First, let's reconnect with your "why." Go back to chapters 1 and 2 and revisit some of the exercises there. Why do you have this book in your hands now? Why are you reading these words? Why haven't you given up, even if what you're doing at this point is just reading and not yet changing?

_____

_____

Second, dig deeper. Think through the change you want to make. How will your life be different? See the Miracle/Magic Question in chapter 4. Capture some of your thoughts.

_____

_____

Third, ground yourself in a small shift that you can easily make. What is one thing you can do today—maybe even right now—that will get you back on your journey again? Try to pick something small enough that you can repeat it easily. This is just a small change to get started on the journey again. For example, when I'm trying to restart my journey, I often start with containing when I eat rather than focusing on what I am eating. It's easier for me to say something like "I will not eat after 7 p.m." rather than dive deeper into what I am eating, which can feel overwhelming at times. Maybe your small shift is even just texting someone in your life who you think can help you on this journey, even something as simple as what Dr. X texted me: "I want to stop working so hard." Or, maybe, your step today is as simple as taking a shower.

_____

_____

Fourth, what might get in the way? Anticipate any challenges. Think about the triggers you captured above. What are some of the hurdles we should be aware of and how can we navigate those challenges to keep you moving forward?

_____

_____

Finally, connect with what you're doing well. When we're feeling "unmotivated," we are often hard on ourselves needlessly. I get it. It makes sense and…step back and look at what *is* working. What are you doing well already (like reading these words for starters)?

_____

_____

We are just getting restarted here and that is okay. That's what this whole book is for…to help you on your imperfect change journey.

Connecting with Your Strengths

As we wrap up this part of the journey, take a look in the proverbial mirror. Let's give yourself some affirmations. When individuals struggle with recurrence, they only see the struggle and forget the strength they have inside themselves. Look at this list of words that describe individuals who have successfully changed their behavior. Circle what you recognize in yourself.

Accepting	Committed	Flexible	Persevering	Stubborn
Active	Competent	Focused	Persistent	Thankful
Adaptable	Concerned	Forgiving	Positive	Thorough
Adventuresome	Confident	Forward-looking	Powerful	Thoughtful
Affectionate	Considerate	Free	Prayerful	Tough
Affirmative	Courageous	Happy	Quick	Trusting
Alert	Creative	Healthy	Reasonable	Trustworthy
Alive	Decisive	Hopeful	Receptive	Truthful

Ambitious	Dedicated	Imaginative	Relaxed	Understanding
Anchored	Determined	Ingenious	Reliable	Unique
Assertive	Die-hard	Intelligent	Resourceful	Unstoppable
Assured	Diligent	Knowledgeable	Responsible	Vigorous
Attentive	Doer	Loving	Sensible	Visionary
Bold	Eager	Mature	Skillful	Whole
Brave	Earnest	Open	Solid	Willing
Bright	Effective	Optimistic	Spiritual	Winning
Capable	Energetic	Orderly	Stable	Wise
Careful	Experienced	Organized	Steady	Worthy
Cheerful	Faithful	Patient	Straight	Zealous
Clever	Fearless	Perceptive	Strong·	Zestful

Now draft some affirmations for yourself. You might have circled "patient" and "strong" and can write something as simple as "I am patient and strong." Or, you can add on "I am patient and strong and will weather this." Make this your own. Affirm what you have inside yourself.

_____

_____

_____

_____

_____

IN YOUR POCKET: Affirmations are an underrated tool. Capture what you wrote above and put it in your pocket. Take a picture of the words, consider posting on social media, record yourself saying the words, whatever it takes to stay connected with who you are and the good you have inside you. And then, in the moment that things get hard or you feel urges you don't want to follow and the harsh voice of self-criticism rising up, use it.

Moving Forward

Here's a recap of what we learned and did in this chapter:

- Reconnected with your original "why" and captured your current "why"

- Learned about how important it is to be mindful of rewards in the behavior change process

- Examined the pros and cons of changing and not changing and consolidated it all into a simple 2x2 grid to help increase your awareness of the forces at play

- Reviewed what triggers are and worked to identify some of your personal triggers, including learning about HALT and self-care

- Covered some ideas and strategies that can help you navigate triggers

- Identified what to do if recurrence of the old behaviors shows up

- Connected with your strengths and worked on self-affirmations

- What else? What are you taking away from this chapter?

_____

_____

_____

That was a lot! And we are almost at the end. In the epilogue, we'll review and consolidate all you have learned in this book and get you ready for the future. Think of the epilogue as discharge planning—we will set you up with a plan for the future so you know how to continue to care for yourself and keep yourself on the path to creating the life you want.

Stepping into a Changed Life

Yesterday I was clever, so I wanted to change the world. Today I am wise, so I am changing myself.

—Rumi, attributed

We did it… And we can do it again if we need to. Here is what is super cool about this book (and about life). You can do it over and over again. You can use it with the same change if your resolve wanes or with a completely different change you find you want to embark on. Change, like life, is a process—not a destination—seriously! So, even though it looks like we're at the end of the book, the book is here so you can go back to any part as often as you need. Flip around to where you need it most. This process doesn't have to be linear. No one is going to judge you. This book in your hands is yours and is intended to be used repeatedly to support your journey.

That said, often patients and I get to the point in our journey together when we feel like we have met our goals and no longer need regular meetings. At that point, we take a step back, consolidate what was learned, and make a plan to identify when a tune-up or refresher is needed. We also take some time to celebrate the gains that have been made, and look ahead to the gains that will be made in the future. If you're game, let's do that together now as you wrap up this journey.

Check Your Pockets

First, check out what's "in your pockets." Go back through the book and flip through to the various times you put something in your pocket. Chapter 1 started it all with a snapshot of your top values. In chapter 2 you put Wise Mind in your pocket. In chapter 3 you put a simple goal in your pocket and then learned how to track it. Chapter 4 had you reflect and take a pic of your DARN-CATs, and chapter 5 had you put your OARS in your pocket. In chapter 6 you selected a wise-minded starting point, and then in chapter 7 you examined triggers and high-risk situations to keep in your pocket. Go back through each chapter and remind yourself of what's in your pockets—what have you learned—and, once you polish those tools, reflect on whether there's anything you want to add, revisit, redo, or relearn. What else might you want in your pocket?

IN YOUR POCKET: This is a make-your-own "in your pocket." Capture what you want to put in your pocket for yourself. Use this space to write about what will help you along your journey.

_____

_____

_____

_____

_____

Similarly, let's take a moment to review the tools in your toolbox, the skills you have picked up or reinforced along the way. What muscles did you strengthen and which ones might need some continued strength building?

We practiced self-compassion all the way back in chapter 1 and mentioned it often in our journey. When is the last time you were kind and gentle to yourself? Consider a Self-Compassion Break right now.

We also worked together on the skills of acceptance (chapter 1) and mindfulness (chapter 3), and we have talked a ton about your values. They are already in your pocket, and there's value (pun intended) to revisiting them often.

EXERCISE: Change Master of the Present

When you visited with the Change Master of the Past, it helped you connect with your strengths and behavioral achievements. Now, let's use this same strategy and check in with your Change Master of the Present. Close your eyes and think: What have you had some success changing in your current journey? What were you able to change? Focus on what worked. You may notice some "yes, but's," assuming your journey wasn't perfect; notice them and bring your mind back to what *did* work, what is different, in a positive direction. If you are willing, close your eyes for a few moments…

Eyes open? Now fill out as much of this as you can and let's look at what you know already:

What behavior(s) did you work on changing in this book?

_____

How similar or different was that change compared to previous changes?

_____

_____

What did *you* do to make the change happen this time? What skills did you leverage? Which "in your pockets" were most helpful?

_____

What worked to support your change this time? _____

Why? _____

What didn't work for you? What might you change going forward? _____

Why? _____

Who were the people in your life who supported your change? _____

How? _____

_____

What did you learn from this last change experience, if you had to boil it all down?

_____

And, in which ways did you knock it out of the park? What parts of this change process would you implement again?

_____

If you could go back to when you started this book and tap yourself on the shoulder, what advice would you give your past self? What would you do differently?

_____

_____

_____

Other insights or observations? Capture those here.

_____

_____

"Warning Signs"

How will you know it's time to come back to the book or to seek additional support? How can you tell whether or not that's something you can get from a friend or family member, and when you need to call in a professional helper such as a mental or physical health care practitioner? Think back to the last chapter, where we reviewed various triggers. Imagine how you can use your awareness muscle to notice when your thoughts, feelings, and behaviors might be slipping back toward your old ways, toward the old status quo, the behaviors you're working on changing. Here are some spots to pay particular attention to for warning signs:

- **Your thoughts—what you say to yourself.** We can't control what you think, and, well, just because you think something doesn't make it true. Join me for a second in a fun demonstration. Put your hands up above your head. Go ahead; raise both hands up high. Now say aloud, with your hands still up, "I can't put my hands above my head. I can't put my hands above my head. I can't put my hands above my head." Wait—your hands are above your head! See, just because you think it, and say it, doesn't make it true. Thoughts can be sneaky and flat out wrong. Thoughts also come and go quickly, often outside our conscious awareness. Raising your attention to what is flowing through your head is important. The behavior change world has a phrase, "stinkin' thinkin'." It's when your thoughts are starting to veer off in a direction that isn't helpful. When you find yourself saying things like *You can have just one* _____ (e.g., beer, potato chip) or *I am a failure* or *I will never succeed*, or when the "f*ck its" show back up, or when you hear yourself say something like *Might as well just give up* after a recurrence, these are all indicators that it's time to double down and get back on track. Similarly, if you notice what we refer to as all/nothing or black/white thinking (thinking at the extremes), that might be a warning sign. Your thoughts often relate to how you might be feeling or what kinds of things you might be doing. So, some stinkin' thinkin' might be about shame, and you might then feel sad or resentful and then choose to avoid activities that are conducive to your behavior change. If you're noticing an abundance of unhelpful, upsetting thoughts that you can't shake with stuff like pleasant activities or distraction, consider getting some outside help. My best advice would be to find someone who is skilled in cognitive behavioral therapy (CBT) and maybe even MI! You deserve to be living your best life, and there are people to help you do that.

- **People, places, things.** Similarly, if you start to notice you're spending more time around people, places, and things you had been avoiding in support of your behavior change, ask yourself what's going on. And, do you have a plan in place for how to deal with triggers? Is your plan strong enough to be around those people, places, or things? Or, conversely, is there something about the change you're working on that might not be working as you originally intended? Maybe it wasn't as in line with your values as you thought? This journey is about creating the life you want to live, and doing that thoughtfully and intentionally will help you stay on the path toward sustained change. When you notice people, places, or things slipping back in *without a plan*, there might be something going on that's worth paying attention to.

What are some warning signs you've noticed in your behavior change journey? And what might you want to be on the lookout for?

_____

_____

_____

Be the Lifeguard of Your Life

When was the last time you were at the pool or beach, or "down the shore" as we say here in New Jersey? Ever watch lifeguards and observe their behavior? They spend their time being vigilant, watching carefully for signs of danger. They're trained to scan the water constantly and mindfully. They know what's risky for swimmers and when they are in trouble. But, even more importantly, they don't sit up on their stands for hours on end. Do you know what they do to keep themselves sharp and maintain their vigilance? They take breaks, they move, they shift with other lifeguards. Know why? A lifeguard is human, just like you and me, and their mind can get bored or habituate (get accustomed) to what they're seeing. To keep their mind, eyes, and body vigilant, they keep it fresh with breaks and changes. Lifeguards also stay in shape and connected with their meaning and purpose—saving lives.

How does this apply to your behavior change journey? Remember our discussion of rewards in chapter 7: we can get tired of or used to what is keeping us engaged, and when that happens, we can lose that motivational oomph without realizing it. So, just like a lifeguard, you have to be aware of what's risky and what's real trouble. You need to work hard to keep your awareness fresh and keep yourself connected with what is important. There are lots of ways you can keep yourself aware, just like the lifeguard. Here are some ideas that you already have onboard:

- **Mindful awareness.** Check in with yourself regularly. Just stop, find your feet, and ask yourself, *How am I doing? What is working? What should I shift? Do I notice any signs of danger or high risk?* Leverage your mindfulness to observe your change talk and your sustain talk. How are you talking to yourself about change? What are your DARN-CATs looking like— are they abundant and strong?

- **Tracking:** Use one of your handy tracking tools in this book to observe whether you're continuing to achieve your goals or not. If you have been tracking and stopped, ask yourself why—sometimes that's an indication that you've gotten bored or offtrack.

- **Ask others for help:** Lifeguards never lifeguard alone. Ask for help from your tribe—the folks in your life who love and care for you. Use your good communication skills from chapter 5 to help them understand how to help you most effectively.

How will you activate your lifeguard skills to be vigilant and keep yourself engaged in your journey? How does that link up to the warning signs you noted above?

Readiness to Change Revisited

In chapter 2 we talked about your readiness to change at the beginning of this journey and reviewed the change categories that people generally fall into (precontemplation, contemplation, preparation, action, recurrence, and maintenance). And here we are getting ready to wrap up your change journey, so let's take a look at where you are right now, in this moment. Consider walking through these three steps to check in with yourself about where you are, give yourself an opportunity to consolidate your motivation, and allow yourself some self-compassion as you walk through the process.

Step 1: Stages of Change Assessment

You might remember the assessment from chapter 2. We talked about how stages of change are states and can shift based on what is going on for you. Often folks move through the stages of change, although not always (not often) in a straight line. You may have started our journey in the contemplation (getting ready) stage and have moved into action with a small detour to recurrence at some point. Or maybe your path has been a little different. This could be a helpful moment to check in with yourself and see where you are to help inform what has or hasn't worked for you in the journey and what you need right now. You can head to http://www.newharbinger.com/51543 and complete the University of Rhode Island Change Assessment (URICA) to determine what stage you're currently in.

Readiness Check Point: What do you make of what stage you're in? How does that compare with where you started? What do you think you could do to move yourself forward or keep yourself engaged in your change journey?

_____

_____

_____

_____

Step 2: Rulers

Earlier in our journey we checked in on the importance of your change to you, your confidence, and your readiness with a set of rulers. Let's leverage those rulers here to help give you a sense of where you are now and how that might compare to where you were previously—again, helping you align with what is or isn't working for you, what you need to keep doing, and what you might need to change.

Importance

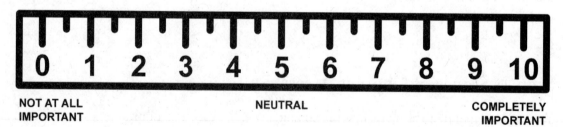

NOT AT ALL   NEUTRAL   COMPLETELY
IMPORTANT   IMPORTANT

Confidence

**NOT AT ALL
CONFIDENT**   **NEUTRAL**   **COMPLETELY
CONFIDENT**

Readiness

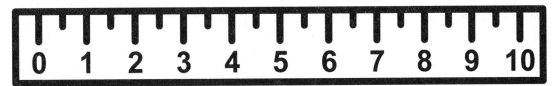

**NOT AT ALL
READY**   **NEUTRAL**   **COMPLETELY
READY**

Readiness Check Point: How do your responses on these rulers compare to your earlier responses? Have you moved forward or backward or remained about the same? What is different for you? Where can you still support movement?

_____

_____

_____

_____

Step 3: Dear Self

This is an opportunity to have a connected conversation with your future self. You can use the space below, grab a piece of paper, or open a doc on your computer or phone if you prefer. My preference for something like this, though, is handwriting. Writing by hand deepens your thought process.

Write a letter to your future self. Capture what areas in your life you have or are trying to impact. Note how you feel or want to feel and what values are at play during this change journey. Use this letter to provide your future self some reminders or advice. This is a chance to take a written snapshot of this moment.

Here's what this might look like for someone on a change journey to be more active and exercise more:

> Hey you,
>
> I really hope this note finds you well. You have worked hard to get yourself on track with exercise. You do SOMEthing every day—even just walking the dogs—and work toward closing your exercise/move rings on your watch even when you don't feel like it. Now you're even training to run your first 5K. It's not always easy, and you figured out how to use friends and family to support your journey. You feel amazing and have more energy than you've had in a long time. You make working out a priority because you see yourself as a priority—something I don't think you could've said about yourself before. Best part? You are having fun. Go you!
>
> If when this letter finds you, you have waivered and aren't on track, find your way back!! This is important stuff. Ask for help—there are plenty of people out there who care about you and will help you get back on track. You have done this once and can do this again.
>
> Always by your side (or inside!),
>
> You

Write your own note to yourself and store it somewhere safe. Set a reminder to open it in a few months (two to three would work), or ask a trusted person to mail it to you later. If you're techy, you can take a pic and email it to yourself with a delay-send. You do what works for you, and tapping your future self on the shoulder in a few months is going to be a meaningful checkpoint.

And that's it! Or, well, it's not *it*. As Winston Churchill once said, "This is not the end, this is not even the beginning of the end, this is just perhaps the end of the beginning." You are on the path to creating the life you want. Keep going. And know that we—you, me, and everyone who's engaged in the project of changing their lives, one step at a time—are all in this together. Thank you for allowing me to join you on this journey.

Acknowledgments

And, when you want something, all the universe conspires in helping you to achieve it.

—Paulo Coelho, *The Alchemist*

If you are reading this, it means you and I both made it this far, and I certainly did not get here alone. The universe has conspired, starting with lots of love and support.

This book would *not have been possible* without the empowerment, collaboration, and inspiration of the amazing Laura A. Saunders.

Thank you to the team at New Harbinger, especially Ryan Buresh, who believed in my vision and encouraged my voice, and Vicraj Gill and Rona Bernstein, who kept my voice in line. I am also grateful to the writing friends who came before me, including Drs. Jill Stoddard, Jack Groppel, Tom Horvath, Amy Bucher, and Ilyse DiMarco, who provided support throughout this journey.

Special thanks to Dr. David Rosengren, who long ago demonstrated the path to make MI accessible and who believed in me enough to agree to write the foreword to this book—an incredible honor I am humbled by.

And to my family for making time and space—Patrick and Natasha, "thank you" are two words that cannot capture the sea of my love and gratitude for all you do to lift me up and help me be the best version of myself, keeping me on my path toward creating the life I want. And, my brother, who has always had my back. Thank you also to my chosen "family," especially Aileen, who answered a call for help to read the final manuscript.

All of my mentors who saw in me what I couldn't see in myself—thank you! Special thanks to the professors of Franklin & Marshall College (Drs. Ricardo Alonso, Jack Heller, and many others); Rutgers, The State University of New Jersey (Drs. Barbara McCrady and Beth Epstein); and University of California, San Diego (Dr. Tammy Wall), who helped this first-generation college student find her way.

Thank you to the CBT Center team who supported me in this endeavor and to my emotional support lawyer and lifelong friend, Shaun Blick.

This book would not have been possible were it not for all the humans over the years who have entrusted their wellbeing and/or their professional training to me. Thank you for working with me and teaching me about the behavior change process.

Finally, a shout-out to the community of evidence-based trainers, supervisors, and clinicians who have inspired me to the greatest heights. An exceptionally warm nod and hug for the MINTie community and fellow MI enthusiasts, including the JJP trio, and Drs. Bill Miller and Steve Rollnick for creating MI and modeling unselfish collaboration. Thank you!

References

Chia, G. L. C., A. Anderson, and L. A. McLean. 2019. "Behavior Change Techniques Incorporated in Fitness Trackers: Content Analysis." *JMIR mHealth and uHealth* 7(7): e12768.

Dozois, D. J., H. A. Westra, K. A. Collins, T. S. Fung, and J. K. Garry. 2004. "Stages of Change in Anxiety: Psychometric Properties of the University of Rhode Island Change Assessment (URICA) Scale." *Behaviour Research and Therapy* 42(6): 711–729.

Drapkin, M. L., P. Wilbourne, J. K. Manuel, J. Baer, B. Karlin, and S. Raffa. 2016. "National Dissemination of Motivation Enhancement Therapy in the Veterans Health Administration: Training Program Design and Initial Outcomes." *Journal of Substance Abuse Treatment* 65: 83–87.

Frost, H., P. Campbell, M. Maxwell, R. E. O'Carroll, S. U. Dombrowski, B. Williams, H. Cheyne, E. Coles, and A. Pollock. 2018. "Effectiveness of Motivational Interviewing on Adult Behaviour Change in Health and Social Care Settings: A Systematic Review of Reviews." *PloS One* 13(10): e0204890.

Gordon, T. n.d. "Origins of the Gordon Model." https://www.gordontraining.com/thomas-gordon/origins-of-the-gordon-model.

Grant, A. Twitter Post. July 28, 2022. https://twitter.com/AdamMGrant/status/15526666 06538481664.

Hardcastle, S. J., M. Fortier, N. Blake, and M. S. Hagger. 2017. "Identifying Content-Based and Relational Techniques to Change Behaviour in Motivational Interviewing." *Health Psychology Review* 11: 1–16.

Harris, R. 2019. *ACT Made Simple: An Easy-to-Read Primer on Acceptance and Commitment Therapy.* Oakland, CA: New Harbinger Publications.

Kabat-Zinn, J. 2003. "Mindfulness-Based Interventions in Context: Past, Present, and Future." *Clinical Psychology: Science and Practice* 10: 144–156.

Kosovski, J. R., and D. C. Smith. 2011. "Everybody Hurts: Addiction, Drama, and the Family in the Reality Television Show *Intervention*." *Substance Use & Misuse* 46: 852–858.

Linehan, M. 2014. *DBT Skills Training Manual*, 2nd ed. New York: Guilford Publications.

Linehan, M. 2021. *Building a Life Worth Living: A Memoir*. New York: Random House.

Michie S, C. Abraham, C. Whittington, J. McAteer, and S. Gupta. 2009. "Effective Techniques in Healthy Eating and Physical Activity Interventions: A Meta-Regression." *Health Psychology* 28: 690–701.

Michie, S., M. M. van Stralen, and R. West. 2011. "The Behaviour Change Wheel: A New Method for Characterising and Designing Behaviour Change Interventions." *Implementation Science* 6: 1–12.

Miller, W. R., A. Zweben, C. C. DiClemente, and R. G. Rychtarik. 1992. "Motivational Enhancement Therapy Manual: A Clinical Research Guide for Therapists Treating Individuals with Alcohol Abuse and Dependence." *Project MATCH Monograph Series* 2. Rockville, MD: National Institute on Alcohol Abuse and Alcoholism.

Miller, W. R., J. C'de Baca, D. B. Matthews, and P. L. Wilbourne. 2001. *Personal Values Card Sort*. University of New Mexico.

Miller, W. R., and S. Rollnick. 2012. *Motivational Interviewing: Helping People Change*. New York: Guilford Press.

Mindful.org. 2022. "Jon Kabat-Zinn: Defining Mindfulness." https://www.mindful.org/jon-kabat-zinn-defining-mindfulness.

Moyers, T. B., T. Martin, P. J. Christopher, J. M. Houck, J. S. Tonigan, and P. C. Amrhein. 2007. "Client Language as a Mediator of Motivational Interviewing Efficacy: Where Is the Evidence?" *Alcoholism: Clinical and Experimental Research* 31: 40s–47s.

Rosengren, D. B. 2017. *Building Motivational Interviewing Skills: A Practitioner Workbook*. New York: Guilford Publications.

Suzuki, S. 2020. *Zen Mind, Beginner's Mind*, 50th anniv. ed. New York: Shambhala Publications.

Michelle L. Drapkin, PhD, ABPP, is a board-certified psychologist who owns and operates the Cognitive Behavioral Therapy Center, and has worked in behavioral science for over twenty years. She held various roles as a behavioral scientist in industry, including leading the development and deployment of behavior change interventions at Johnson & Johnson. She held a national motivational interviewing (MI) training position at the Department of Veterans Affairs (VA), and was on faculty at the University of Pennsylvania. Drapkin completed her PhD in clinical psychology from Rutgers, The State University of New Jersey; and joined the Motivational Interviewing Network of Trainers (MINT) in 2008. She has trained thousands of health care professionals and industry leaders in MI.

Real change *is* possible

For more than forty-five years, New Harbinger has published proven-effective self-help books and pioneering workbooks to help readers of all ages and backgrounds improve mental health and well-being, and achieve lasting personal growth. In addition, our spirituality books offer profound guidance for deepening awareness and cultivating healing, self-discovery, and fulfillment.

Founded by psychologist Matthew McKay and Patrick Fanning, New Harbinger is proud to be an independent, employee-owned company. Our books reflect our core values of integrity, innovation, commitment, sustainability, compassion, and trust. Written by leaders in the field and recommended by therapists worldwide, New Harbinger books are practical, accessible, and provide real tools for real change.

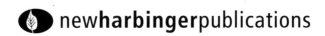 **newharbinger**publications

MORE BOOKS from
NEW HARBINGER PUBLICATIONS

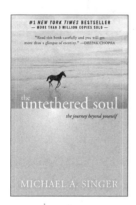

THE UNTETHERED SOUL

The Journey Beyond Yourself

978-1572245372 / US $18.95

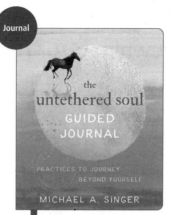

**THE UNTETHERED SOUL
GUIDED JOURNAL**

Practices to Journey Beyond Yourself

978-1684036561 / US $25.95

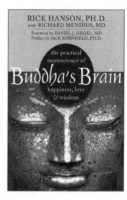

BUDDHA'S BRAIN

The Practical Neuroscience of
Happiness, Love, and Wisdom

978-1572246959 / US $18.95

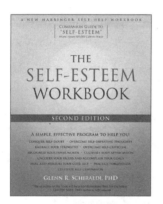

**THE SELF-ESTEEM
WORKBOOK,
SECOND EDITION**

978-1626255937 / US $22.95

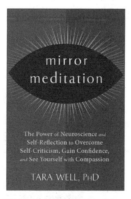

MIRROR MEDITATION

The Power of Neuroscience and
Self-Reflection to Overcome
Self-Criticism, Gain Confidence, and
See Yourself with Compassion

978-1684039678 / US $17.95

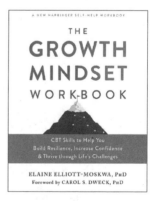

**THE GROWTH MINDSET
WORKBOOK**

CBT Skills to Help You Build
Resilience, Increase Confidence, and
Thrive through Life's Challenges

978-1684038299 / US $24.95

new harbinger publications

1-800-748-6273 / newharbinger.com

(VISA, MC, AMEX / prices subject to change without notice)
Follow Us

Did you know there are **free tools** you can download for this book?

Free tools are things like **worksheets**, **guided meditation exercises**, and **more** that will help you get the most out of your book.

You can download free tools for this book—whether you bought or borrowed it, in any format, from any source—from the New Harbinger website. All you need is a NewHarbinger.com account. Just use the URL provided in this book to view the free tools that are available for it. Then, click on the "download" button for the free tool you want, and follow the prompts that appear to log in to your NewHarbinger.com account and download the material.

You can also save the free tools for this book to your **Free Tools Library** so you can access them again anytime, just by logging in to your account! Just look for this button on the book's free tools page.

+ Save this to my free tools library

If you need help accessing or downloading free tools, visit **newharbinger.com/faq** or contact us at **customerservice@newharbinger.com**.